NOURISH
Your Noggin

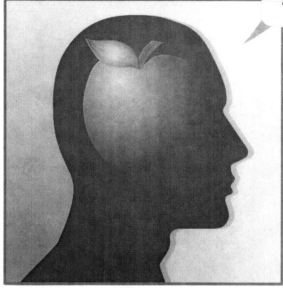

Brain-Building Foods and **Easy-To-Make Recipes** To
Hasten Your Healing From Mild Traumatic Brain Injury
(Concussion & Post Concussion Syndrome)

Tina M. Sullivan

Integrative Heath & Nutrition Coach, AADP

Outskirts Press, Inc.
Denver, Colorado

Nourish Your Noggin
Brain-Building Foods & Easy-to-Make Recipes to Hasten Your Healing From Mild Traumatic Brain Injury (Concussion & Post Concussion Syndrome)

Outskirts Press, Inc.
http://www.outskirtspress.com

ISBN: 978-1-4327-7895-8

Outskirts Press and the "OP" logo are trademarks belonging to Outskirts Press, Inc.

PRINTED IN THE UNITED STATES OF AMERICA

WHAT PEOPLE ARE SAYING ABOUT
NOURISH YOUR NOGGIN

"In 1990, when I sustained my traumatic brain injury, there was virtually no information about how foods could affect your brain or brain recovery. The hypoglycemia diet was the only one that mentioned how it can affect brain clarity and brain fog. As a board certified health Psychologist and Neuropsychologist, I knew then that what you ate did affect your brain. Tina Sullivan's expertise in nutrition as an Integrative Health and Nutrition Coach has provided you, the reader, with a book written with love that provides knowledge of brain injury, how and why food affects the brain and some really wonderful menus."

Dr. Diane Roberts Stoler, Ed.D.
Licensed Psychologist
Board Certified Health Psychologist
Board Certified Sport Psychologist
Neuropsychologist
Author: *Coping with Mild Traumatic Brain Injury*

"Tina Sullivan's Nourish Your Noggin could not be a more welcome book for our military medical providers and families. Military personnel serving in combat zones know only too well how devastating blasts can be. Less obvious and harder to understand are the long-term effects of the shock wave on the brain. Just shy of 2 million U.S. military personnel have deployed to Iraq or Afghanistan since the start of military operations in 2001 with Traumatic Brain Injury (TBI) or concussion as one of the most common forms of combat-related injury. These injuries may go undiagnosed and untreated for days, months, or years as attention is focused on the more "visible" injuries. Nourish Your Noggin brings a real awareness to TBI, helps you walk through health care choices, and gives you healthy food choices for a well-nourished brain.

This book is a must read!"

Colonel (Retired) Mike Santacroce
USMC
OIF/OEF Veteran
Bronze Star

"Since I started The Healthy Brain Program© in Canada, over 10 years ago, people have been asking me about what is the best kind of food for the brain. The quick answer is, 'a Mediterranean-type diet.' However, there is a subgroup of patients, those who have suffered head injury and who are always interested in what more they can do to optimize their brain function and quality of life. To this population, you have delivered a terrific service. Your advice is germane and easy to follow with good backup of reference materials.

You were able to 'fine tune' the usual healthy diet to this population with even more specific needs! I believe it will be complementary to your work and website, and it will be of great benefit to those who wish to follow healthy nutrition principles.

I also love your recipes. I did not realize that brown rice could be that good! Having read your book has made me look at my own nutrition again, and I was able to weed out some useless foods. Thank you for your dedicated effort on this usually ignored topic."

Kind regards,

Stephen J. Kiraly, MD, FRCPC, ABPN,
Clinical Associate Professor, Faculty of Medicine, University of British Columbia, Department of Psychiatry, Division of Geriatric Psychiatry, Consultant, Geriatric Psychiatry, Vancouver Coastal Health Authority, Canada.

TABLE OF CONTENTS

This book is dedicated to my son, Shane, whose bravery, courage and sense of humor have consistently amazed me and reinforced my belief that God gives us the "tools" to deal with tragedy and daily trials with grace and hope.

FOREWORD

Until recently, the concept of nutrition was on the back burner, and it was not a part of the medical community training unless someone had diabetes or heart problems. Only then, in these situations, was a person with either of these conditions given a special diet or nutritional counseling. However, to the general population, what we ate was hardly of any concern. Retailers then realized that they could sell more products if they linked proper nutrition with physical disease. Only in the past decade have we seen advertisements geared to eat nutritious foods for your heart.

Along with this trend, First Lady Mrs. Obama has a campaign for obesity in America that now includes newer nutritional packaging and encouragement of eating for a healthier physical being. Along with this has come the concept of brain food or eating food that will help you with your memory.

In 1990, when I sustained my traumatic brain injury, there was virtually no information about how foods could affect your brain or brain recovery. The hypoglycemia diet was the only one that mentioned how it can affect brain clarity and brain fog.

As a board certified health psychologist and neuropsychologist, I knew then that what you ate did affect your brain. From this knowledge, I took the current information at the time of my brain injury and experimented with the hypoglycemic diet and what was the then food pyramid. From there, I developed a brain diet for myself and the patients I've worked with since—most of whom call my program the "diet from hell," because I did not have the nutritional background or culinary arts to suggest what menu they could put together for a brain diet that was both nutritious and enjoyable to eat.

This book provides the bridge and essential information for both. Throughout this book, you are provided with the nutritional aspects of eating healthy along with menus that you will look forward to using.

This book is written by a mother with first-hand knowledge of my diet, seeing how it has worked for her son, Shane's, brain injury. Tina Sullivan's expertise in nutrition as an Integrative Health and Nutrition Coach has provided you, the reader, with a book written with love that provides knowledge of brain injury, how and why food affects the brain, and some really wonderful menus.

Warmest Regards,

Dr. Diane Roberts Stoler, Ed.D.
Licensed Psychologist
Board Certified Health Psychologist
Board Certified Sport Psychologist
Neuropsychologist
Author: Coping with Mild Traumatic Brain Injury

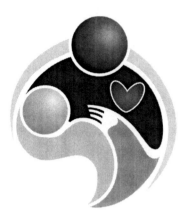

"Before you can inspire with emotion, you must be swamped with it yourself. Before you can move their tears, your own must flow. To convince them, you must yourself believe." –
Winston Churchill

PREFACE
Our Story

In May of 2010, my 13-year-old son, Shane, was away for the weekend with some friends. The first night that they were there, he was playing a game and tripped over a friend's foot. He fell backwards and slammed the back of his head on the wood floor full force. He got up, felt a little disoriented and dizzy, but he was conscious. He sat down with a friend's mom and tried to ride out the immediate symptoms, but he still felt a little "out of it." That night, he experienced a severe headache and nausea, but he was able to sleep it off. Extremely relieved to be feeling better the next morning, Shane was able to function normally for the rest of the weekend. He did not see a doctor at this time.

Aside from periodic dizziness and a little confusion in the weeks that followed, my son was able to participate fully at school, at home, and with friends. A MONTH & A HALF LATER, while Shane was at a friend's house playing badminton, he returned a shot and suddenly fell to his knees. This seemingly innocent fall was enough to shake his brain and disrupt his brain tissue and brain function. This event was the straw that broke the camel's back. Within the hour, he had lines in his vision and echoed hearing, and he felt very scared and disoriented. He called his dad to pick him up "NOW."

I was away at a conference in NYC and was to return the following day. My husband calmed my son and checked on him several times throughout the night to make sure that he was ok. The next morning, he was examined by the primary doctor on call. The doctor did not think that any of his symptoms were related to the concussion in May, and he sent him home to rest and take it easy. However, this time, the symptoms did not go away; they got much worse. Thus, began Shane's journey into the scary world of "Mild Traumatic Brain Injury" AND "Post Concussion Syndrome."

Our lives STOPPED. The blessing was that it was school vacation, and we did not have to think about him missing school. The very difficult part was watching our child experiencing severe neurological symptoms that were scary and overwhelming.

All at once he was dealing with the following side effects from the head injury:

- Confusion

- Dizziness

- Episodes of vertigo

- Couldn't watch TV, look at a computer, and play video or Wii games

- Extreme sensitivity to light and sound

- Pressure headaches that lasted all day and into the night

- Debilitating waves of anxiety & emotion

- And many other symptoms

Along with having him evaluated by a Pediatric Neurologist at Children's Hospital in Boston, I continued to do the two other things I knew I could do: pray and become his advocate by researching the best proactive steps we could take to help him to heal as quickly and fully as his brain would allow.

This research led us to working with Dr. Diane Roberts Stoler, a brilliant Neuropsychologist specializing in Neurofeedback who has sustained several Traumatic Brain Injuries herself and has fully recovered. She now helps others around the country heal from their own brain injuries, including Shane.

As an Integrative Health and Nutrition Coach, I fully understood that the foods that Shane was eating could positively or negatively affect his brain's ability to heal. Dr. Diane Roberts Stoler agreed, and in fact, she provides specific dietary guidelines for her patients.

This is where our family's personal journey with MTBI and my nutritional coaching experience come together to serve you. As a mom of another child with several food allergies, I already knew how to research, shop for, and cook for our family "outside the box." Shane's new dietary restrictions required me to take it up a couple of notches. Even though it was tough, this was doable for me.

I fully understand that dealing with and recovering from a Mild Traumatic Brain Injury is very overwhelming by itself for you and your family, friends, and colleagues. This book was created as a practical guide about what you should eat while you are healing so that you don't have to figure it out on your own!

This book will teach you:

- What foods to avoid so that you don't hinder your body's ability to heal.

- What foods to eat and enjoy so that you can promote health and sustained energy.

- Recipes that taste great and are not complicated to prepare.

- Where to locate ingredients and healthy meals when you don't feel like cooking.

- Other helpful websites and resources.

I am honored to share this knowledge with you. I hope that this book will be a helpful tool as you navigate your path of healing from your brain injury.

Wishing you the best,

Tina M. Sullivan
Integrative Health & Nutrition Coach, AADP

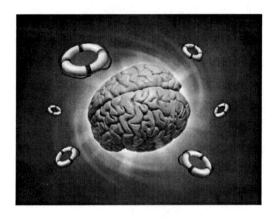

"Nothing can happen through you until it happens to you, and you can only communicate what you're in the process of rediscovering." – Lloyd John Ogilvie

CHAPTER I

A Quick Review of Mild Traumatic Brain Injury & Post Concussion Syndrome

The brain is the most important organ in the body. It is soft in consistency like jelly, and it sits in a bony cranium with jagged outcroppings and membranes that support it so that it does not collapse onto itself. This softness and strange architecture is why the brain is so vulnerable to injury.

Traumatic Brain Injury is a very common neurological disorder affecting 180 people out of every 100,000. The most recent studies done by the CDC indicate that 1.7 million people sustain a Traumatic Brain Injury in the US annually. About 15% of people who suffer a TBI will be permanently symptomatic. Recent reports estimate that 5.3 million or around 2% of the US population live with disabilities resulting from a Traumatic Brain Injury.

Symptoms resulting from a Traumatic Brain Injury can be mild, moderate, or severe. However, these terms have nothing to do with the severity of the injury.

Mild Traumatic Brain Injury Defined

Mild Traumatic Brain Injury (MTBI) is the result of the forceful motion of the head or impact to the head, causing a brief change in mental status, (confusion, disorientation, or loss of memory) or loss of consciousness for less than 60 minutes. About 80% of TBI's are classified as "mild," using the Glasgow Coma Scale. Mild Traumatic Brain Injury affects about 1,000,000 Americans every year. These injuries most commonly occur due to car accidents (45%), falls (30%), occupational accidents (10%), recreational accidents (10%), and assault (5%).

Mild Traumatic Brain Injury is often missed at the time of the initial injury. Other terms commonly used to describe MTBI are:

- Concussion,

- Minor head trauma,

- Minor TBI,

- Minor brain injury,

- Minor head injury, or

- Post concussion syndrome.

The word concussion comes from the Latin word *concutere* which means "to shake violently." In 2004, the Second International Conference on Concussion classified concussions into two categories: "simple" and "complex." When a person suffers a simple concussion, it resolves without any complications within 7-10 days by limiting activity and resting. A complex concussion is more serious and the individual usually suffers ongoing symptoms.

According to Dr. Stephen J. Kiraly, MD, FRCPC, in his book, *Your Healthy Brain*, "All concussions mandate evaluation by a doctor and must be diagnosed and graded, and the appropriate concussion management protocol should be applied." The Sports Concussion Assessment Tool (SCAT) was developed by a group of neuropsychiatrists and neurosurgeons to help coaches, teachers, and athletes in medically evaluating concussions. You can find this helpful tool through the links at Dr. Kiraly's website: www. healthybrain.org, or you can google: "Sports Concussion Assessment Tool" for more in depth information.

In Dr. Diane Roberts Stoler's book, *Coping with Mild Traumatic Brain Injury*, it is stated, "There are two forms of MTBI: direct contact force and diffuse." Direct contact force results in observable tissue damage to a particular area of the brain. This can occur during a car accident or when the forward-moving head comes to a sudden stop after striking a stationary object. When this happens, the brain keeps moving within the skull until it makes sudden contact with the front of the inner skull. This causes bruising of the frontal and/ or temporal lobes of the brain. A second type of direct contact force MTBI is the coup/contrecoup injury which occurs when a moving object makes contact with the head, briefly denting the skull inward. The brain beneath the dent is bruised first, and then it is thrown against the opposite side of the skull where additional bruising takes place.

A diffuse MTBI is described as a mild blow to the head that causes momentary unconsciousness but no observable disruption of nerve impulses. It was originally believed that diffuse MTBI's caused only a brief short-circuiting within the brain. However, Dr. Diane Roberts Stoler writes, "It is now known that the stretching of nerve cells due to movement of the brain in various directions at once interferes with their ability to fire impulses." Diffuse MTBI can happen alone or in conjunction with a direct contact force MTBI.

Mild Traumatic Brain Injury can also result from the following secondary causes:

- Anoxia – lack of oxygen

- Contusion – a bruise that may go undetected during regular testing

- Edema – swelling due to fluid buildup in the brain tissue

- Hematoma – localized brain swelling due to an accumulation of blood from a broken blood vessel

- Hemorrhage – bleeding into the brain tissue from a torn blood vessel

Post Concussion Syndrome

Approximately 40% of MTBI victims develop a cluster of symptoms referred to as Post Concussion Syndrome. They may present as the following:

Type of Symptom	Examples
Physical	Fatigue Sleep disturbances Headaches Dizziness Nausea and vomiting Blurred vision Hearing problems Loss of sex drive
Cognitive (mental)	Distractibility Disorientation Temporary amnesia Short-term memory problems Poor judgment Slow thinking
Emotional	Depression Agitation Apathy Irritability
Behavioral	Confrontational attitude Explosive temper Fearfulness Impatience Thoughtlessness
Secondary psychological	Anxiety and/or Fear of "going crazy" Frustration or anger Guilt or shame Feelings of helplessness

Table 1.1 – *Coping with Mild Traumatic Brain Injury*, Dr. Diane Stoler, Ed.D

Some of the MTBI symptoms of individuals resolve within a few weeks of the injury. 15% of patients have symptoms that persist for a year or more. According to Dr. Stephen Kiraly, MD, (*Your Healthy Brain*) and Dr. Diane Roberts Stoler, Ed.D (*Coping with Mild Traumatic Brain Injury*), the outlook for recovery from MTBI is brightest with early diagnosis and treatment of symptoms. Even if the patient "looks fine," they may need a neuropsychological workup—a diagnostic process designed to reveal problems with reasoning, memory, and other brain functions—to finally pinpoint the source or sources of their difficulties.

Chronic Traumatic Encephalopathy

Chronic Traumatic Encephalopathy is a progressive degenerative disease of the brain that is found in athletes and others who have sustained repetitive brain trauma. This trauma, which is the result of multiple concussions, triggers progressive degeneration of the brain tissue. This creates the build-up of an abnormal protein called tau. These changes in the brain can occur months, years, or even decades after the last concussion. The brain degeneration is associated with memory loss, confusion, impaired judgment, paranoia, impulse control problems, aggression, depression, and, later on, progressive dementia.

Initially referred to as "punch drunk" as early as 1928, it was thought to affect only boxers with symptoms such as speech problems, slowed movement, tremors, and confusion. Through 2009, there were only 49 documented cases of Chronic Traumatic Encephalopathy, 39 of which were boxers. However, in the last decade, a Pittsburg medical examiner, Bennet Omalu, diagnosed two Pittsburg Steelers with the condition—both of whom passed away in 2002 and 2005 respectively.

The Sports Legacy Institute, run by Chris Nowinski and Dr. Robert Cantu, partnered with Drs. Ann McKee and Robert Stern to create the Center for the Study of Traumatic Encephalopathy (CSTE) at the Boston University School of Medicine. In CSTE's first twelve months, they identified CTE in 17 out of 18 deceased contact sports athletes between the ages of 18 and 83. Because of these findings, there is grave concern that CTE affects more athletes than originally believed. For more in depth information, check out http://www.bu.edu/cste/ and http://www.sportslegacy.org/.

I highly recommend Dr. Diane Roberts Stoler's book, *Coping with Mild Traumatic Brain Injury* (available at http://www.health-helper.com/) and Dr. Steven Kiraly's book, *Your Healthy Brain – A Personal & Family Guide to Staying Healthy & Living Longer* (available at healthybrain.org). These books contain a wealth of information not only for the victims of a MTBI but for their families as well as clinical practitioners.

Because MTBI is an injury with so many symptoms that cannot be seen, it was extremely helpful for me to fully understand exactly what my son, Shane, was experiencing on a daily basis. From the summer of 2010 through February of 2011, he has suffered 3 severe concussions (not through sports). Being his constant advocate, I have learned more about Neurology in the last year than I ever thought I would learn in my lifetime. I have also thoroughly researched (and Shane has participated in) many useful therapies that were proactive steps that we could take to hasten his healing without nasty side effects. Sinking my teeth deep into this research enabled me to be empathetic and to provide him with the appropriate support and tools as they were needed.

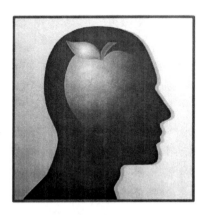

"Knowledge will forever govern ignorance; and a people who mean to be their own governors must arm themselves with the power which knowledge gives." – James Madison

CHAPTER 2
Nutrition & Your Brain

Your body is absolutely amazing! Nerve signals travel through your muscles at almost 200 miles per hour. Your brain can light a 20-watt light bulb with the electric energy it puts out when it is functioning well. Your separate body systems work together synergistically, coordinating millions of tasks and functions every day.

What you eat greatly influences your body's ability to function well. The foods that you eat and drinks that you choose affect you on a cellular level and become your blood, muscles, organs (<u>your brain being the biggest and most important one!</u>), skin, hair, and even your moods. As you have probably heard before, food is "fuel." This "fuel" contains nutrients. Nutrients come in the form of vitamins, minerals, enzymes, water, amino acids, carbohydrates, and lipids. Nutrients do everything from combating infection to repairing tissue to helping you to think.

If you make food choices that are comprised of lots of processed food and drive-thru bargains, then your body's nutritional needs are not being met. A deficiency in good nutrients will impair your body's normal tasks and can cause body parts to malfunction and break down. How well your body is working can be seen in observing your brain function, memory, skin elasticity, eyesight, energy, the ratio of lean to fat tissue in the body, and an overall feeling of well-being.

Brain chemicals called neurotransmitters that regulate your behavior are controlled by the food and beverages that you choose to take in. Neurotransmitters are responsible for your moods. The most commonly known neurotransmitters are dopamine, serotonin, and norepinephrine. When you eat foods that increase serotonin, you become less tense. When the brain creates more dopamine and norepinephrine, you act and think clearer and are more alert.

Why are these neurotransmitters so crucial? They are responsible for relaying impulses between your nerve cells. If you don't have enough serotonin, it can lead to depression, anxiety, and disturbed sleep. When you eat a diet rich in complex carbohydrates (like whole grains, veggies, and fruits), it raises the amino acid, tryptophan. Consuming foods containing tryptophan elevates the level of serotonin in the brain, which in turn calms you down. When you eat good quality, high protein foods (like grass-fed meats, free-range eggs, quinoa, etc.), you increase the levels of dopamine and norepinephrine in your body keeping you alert and present.

Depression can be one of the unfortunate side effects after suffering a Mild Traumatic Brain Injury. One of the most common types of depression is a chronic underlying depression called dysthymia. It includes long-term and recurring depression symptoms that don't necessary disable you, but they do keep you from functioning normally and can interfere with enjoying your life. Arming your food arsenal with healthy choices that combat depression may help keep these symptoms under control.

A brain-healthy diet consists of water, carbohydrates, proteins, fats, vitamins, minerals, and micronutrients. It may sound like a mouthful, but let me break it down into usable components for you. I'll quickly highlight the major categories: water, carbohydrates, proteins, and fats. Then I will show you the essential vitamins and minerals; how they support brain health; and how a deficiency in each compromises brain function. <u>Note: When I discuss vitamins and minerals, I will refer only to how these relate to brain health and body healing, even though each vitamin and mineral mentioned may benefit other functions in the body.</u>

Vitamins & Minerals

All of the vitamins and minerals that I mention here should be first taken in through a varied, whole-foods diet. The information contained here is not intended as a substitute for consulting with your physician. If you choose to add supplements to your diet, please discuss it first with your doctor.

Vitamins

Vitamins are very important. They help to regulate the metabolism and the biochemical processes that release the energy from food that has been digested. Enzymes are catalysts (activators) in the constant chemical reactions that are always happening in the body. Vitamins work with these enzymes to make sure all of the actions are carried out in the body according to plan.

- **Vitamin A**

  Vitamin A strengthens the immune system, and is needed for the maintenance and repair of epithelial tissue. It aids in fat storage, acts as an antioxidant, and is necessary for new cell growth. Protein cannot be used in the body without Vitamin A. The carotenoids are a group of compounds related to Vitamin A. They are beta-carotene, alpha and gamma carotene, and lycopene. Beta-carotene is the best source through the diet, because the liver converts only the amount that the body actually needs—thus, preventing toxicity. Deficiencies in Vitamin A may be insomnia, fatigue, and night blindness. If you have diabetes or hypothyroidism, your body may not be able to convert beta-carotene into Vitamin A.

- **Vitamin B Complex**

  B vitamins maintain healthy nerves, proper brain function and healthy muscle tone. They assist enzymes in their chemical reactions and with energy production. Let's break them down.

- **B1/Thiamine**

  B1 helps with blood formation and circulation. It maximizes cognitive activity and brain function. It affects energy, growth, appetite, and learning ability. Thiamine deficiency symptoms may be fatigue, forgetfulness, irritability, nervousness, numbness, pain and sensitivity, poor coordination, and tingling. Antibiotics, Dilantin (a seizure drug), sulfa drugs, heavy alcohol or caffeine intake may decrease thiamine in the body.

- **B2/Riboflavin**

B2 is helpful with red blood cell creation, antibody production, and growth. It assists with metabolizing carbohydrates, fats, and proteins. Deficiencies may be seen as dizziness, insomnia, and slowed mental response. B2 absorption is affected by antibiotics and alcohol.

- **B3/Niacin**

B3 is used for optimal nervous system functioning and proper circulation. It is helpful for memory enhancement. Symptoms of B3 deficiency include dementia, depression, dizziness, fatigue, headaches, insomnia, muscular weakness, and inflammation.

- **B5/Panothenic Acid**

B5 is considered the "anti-stress vitamin." It is used for the production of adrenal hormones, the formation of antibodies, and to convert fats, carbohydrates, and proteins into energy. It helps to produce neurotransmitters and is a stamina enhancer. It may be helpful for treating depression and anxiety. If you don't have enough B5, you may suffer from fatigue, headaches, and tingling in the hands.

- **B6/Pyridoxine**

B6 is involved in multiple bodily functions and affects both mental and physical health. It helps to absorb fats and proteins and maintains the appropriate sodium and potassium balance. It is crucial for a healthy nervous system, normal brain function, and cellular growth. B6 deficiency may result in convulsions, headaches, depression, dizziness, fatigue, hyper-irritability, learning difficulties and impaired memory, numbness, and tingling. Antidepressants, diuretics, and cortisone drugs can reduce absorption of B6.

- **B12/Cyanocobalamin**

B12 helps folic acid form red blood cells and use iron properly. It's needed for the absorption of foods and the synthesizing of proteins. It helps with forming cells and their longevity. It promotes nerve growth and development because it maintains the fatty sheaths that cover and protect nerve endings. It has been linked to the production of acetylcholine, a neurotransmitter that enables memory and learning. It may also help you to sleep more soundly. B12 deficiency may be seen as chronic fatigue, depression, dizziness, drowsiness, eye disorders, headaches (including migraines), irritability, memory loss, nervousness, neurological damage, ringing in the ears, and spinal cord degeneration. Anti-gout medications, anticoagulant drugs, and potassium supplements may affect absorption. You need "intrinsic factor" (which is a protein produced in the digestive tract) to properly absorb B12.

- **Choline**

Choline is important for nerve impulses to be transmitted effectively from the brain through the central nervous system. Without it, brain function and memory can be impaired. It helps with fat and cholesterol metabolism. Choline deficiency may appear as cardiac symptoms, high blood pressure, and an inability to digest fats.

- **Vitamin C**

Vitamin C is an antioxidant that is utilized by over 300 different functions in the body. It helps with tissue growth and repair and the production of anti-stress hormones, and it binds with and eliminates heavy metals from the body. It protects against abnormal blood clotting and bruising, promotes wound healing, and helps to form collagen. Vitamin C deficiency can result in a susceptibility to infection, lack of energy, and prolonged wound healing time. Alcohol, analgesics, antidepressants, anticoagulants, steroids, and smoking may reduce levels of Vitamin C in the body.

- **Vitamin D3**

Vitamin D3 is considered the most natural and most active form of Vitamin D. It is recognized as a vitamin and a hormone. It is important for proper growth and development, protecting the body against muscle weakness, and it is necessary for normal blood clotting. D2 is obtained through food sources, but it is not active until it is converted by the liver and the kidneys. Vitamin D deficiency may be seen as symptoms such as a lack of appetite, insomnia, and vision problems. Most people living in the upper third of the US are deficient due to lack of sun exposure in the winter. Some cholesterol-lowering drugs, antacids, and steroid hormones (like cortisone) interfere with Vitamin D absorption.

- **Vitamin E**

Vitamin E improves circulation, helps repair tissue, promotes healing, and maintains healthy nerves and muscles. Deficiency may appear as damage to red blood cells and neuromuscular problems. Your body needs zinc to keep Vitamin E up to the correct levels.

- **Folic Acid/Folate**

Folate is referred to as a brain food. It is also used in the formation of red blood cells and the production of energy. As a coenzyme to DNA and RNA synthesis, it is crucial for cell division and replication. It helps to metabolize protein and may help relieve anxiety and depression. Possible neurological signs of folate deficiency are fatigue, growth impairment, insomnia, memory problems, and weakness. Alcohol also can stand in the way of proper folate absorption.

- **Vitamin K**

Vitamin K is used for proper blood clotting. It is also crucial for bone formation and repair and for converting glucose into glycogen for storage. If deficient, you may experience abnormal or internal bleeding. Antibiotics interfere with absorption.

Minerals

You need minerals for your body fluids to be in correct balance, for proper bone and blood formation, and to maintain healthy nerve function and muscle tone. Minerals work as coenzymes, promoting healthy energy, growth, and healing. Each mineral in the body works synergistically with other minerals, so if one is out of balance, the others are affected.

- **Calcium**

Among many other functions, calcium helps to maintain a regular heartbeat and properly transmit nerve impulses. It is used in the protein formation of RNA and DNA, and it aids in neuromuscular activity. Deficiency may be seen as insomnia, muscle cramps, nervousness, numbness, cognitive impairment, depression and hyperactivity. Antacids like Tums are not the best source of calcium, because in order to take in the amount of calcium necessary through this method, the stomach acid needed for the absorption of calcium would be neutralized. Phenobarbital and diuretics may cause a deficiency in calcium.

- **Iron**

Iron produces hemoglobin and oxygenates red blood cells. It is important for growth, a healthy immune system, and energy production. Deficiency can be caused by excessive exercise, insufficient intake, poor digestion, or excessive coffee or tea consumption. Symptoms may appear as dizziness, fatigue, nervousness, and slowed mental reactions. You need sufficient amounts of hydrochloric acid in the stomach for proper absorption of iron.

- **Magnesium**

Magnesium is a catalyst for energy production and helps with calcium and potassium uptake. Taking in magnesium through your diet helps to prevent depression, dizziness, and muscle twitching. It relaxes tight muscles, and it helps to maintain proper pH balance and normal body temperature. A deficiency in magnesium leads to interference with muscle and nerve impulses that may cause irritability and nervousness. Magnesium deficiency may be responsible for confusion, insomnia, irritability, tantrums, and rapid heartbeat. It can also be seen as chronic fatigue, chronic pain syndromes, and depression. It is at the root of many cardiovascular problems. To test for deficiency, a procedure called an intracellular magnesium screen should be performed. Alcohol, diuretics, and high levels of zinc and Vitamin D increase the need for magnesium.

- **Manganese**

Manganese is needed in small amounts for metabolizing proteins and fats, healthy nerves, a healthy immune system, and regulating levels of blood sugar. It is used in the formation of cartilage and the synovial fluid in the joints. It complements the B complex vitamins in creating a feeling of well-being. A deficiency in manganese is very rare.

- **Potassium**

Potassium is needed for a healthy nervous system as well as maintaining a regular heart rhythm. It assists sodium in creating a healthy water balance in the body. It aids in transmitting electrochemical impulses, helps to prevent stroke, and enables muscles to contract efficiently. It also manages the exchange of nutrients through the cell membranes. Deficiency symptoms may include cognitive impairment, depression, reduced reflex function, nervousness, glucose intolerance, growth impairment, insomnia, muscle fatigue, and occasional headaches. Stress, tobacco, and caffeine reduce potassium absorption in the body.

- **Zinc**

Zinc is needed for protein synthesis and for the formation of cartilage. It also helps to maintain a healthy immune system and to heal wounds. It enhances the senses of taste and smell. An adequate intake and retention of zinc in the body is needed to maintain proper levels of Vitamin E. A zinc deficiency may contribute to the loss of taste and smell. It may also manifest as fatigue, diminished ability to see at night, memory loss, and the slow healing of wounds.

Water

Your body is two-thirds water. Water is utilized in every function of the body and transports nutrients and waste out of every single cell. It maintains proper body temperature and is needed for all digestive actions, circulatory functions and for proper absorption of nutrients.

Carbohydrates

Carbohydrates supply your body with the energy it needs to function. They are found in fruits, vegetables, peas, and beans. Milk is the only animal product where carbohydrates can be found. There are simple and complex carbohydrates—complex being the best for you. Simple carbohydrates include fruits (fructose), table sugar (sucrose), milk sugar (lactose), and other simple sugars. Refined sugars—like the ones in soda, candy, and many desserts—are so processed that they contain no beneficial nutrients. Fruit is the only sugar of the "simple" group that your body should be taking in after a Mild Traumatic Brain Injury. (Why? This will be discussed in depth in later chapters.) Complex carbohydrates also include fiber and starches.

Carbohydrates are the main contributor to blood glucose, which is responsible for energizing all of your body's cells. It is also the only source of energy for your brain and red blood cells. This glucose provides energy immediately to the cells or is stored in the liver to be used later.

Proteins

Proteins are critical for growth and development, provide the body with energy, and help with the formation of hormones, antibodies, enzymes and tissues. When you eat protein, your body breaks it down into amino acids. These are the building blocks of all proteins. Your body is able to manufacture "nonessential" amino acids from other amino acids. "Essential" amino acids must be brought into your body through the foods that you eat. Many amino acid combinations are needed to build muscle, for example. If you are deficient in "essential" amino acids for a period of time, your body will stop building protein, compromising your body's ability to heal and function properly.

Complete proteins contain a large array of essential amino acids and are found in meat, fish, poultry, cheese, eggs and milk. Incomplete proteins, which contain only some essential amino acids, are found in grains, legumes, and leafy green vegetables. This doesn't give you a ticket to "pass" on these foods – it just means that you have eat a balance of foods from the two groups for the maximum benefit.

Fats

Your body needs fat; it's important for normal brain development and is essential for providing energy. It is the most concentrated form of energy available to the body. Understanding fats does not have to be overwhelming and confusing! There are five kinds of fatty acids: saturated, polyunsaturated, monounsaturated, trans-fatty acids, and essential fatty acids.

1. Saturated Fatty Acids

These are found primarily in animal products, including meats, dairy products, and vegetable shortening. The marbling that is seen in a cut of meat is saturated fat. Most people eat too much saturated fat, which contributes to high cholesterol in the body. However, there are some saturated fats that are good for you in moderation. (This will be discussed in detail in the "Healthy Fats" section.)

2. Polyunsaturated Fatty Acids

These lower LDL cholesterol and raise HDL cholesterol. They are found in corn oil, soybean oil, safflower oil, sunflower oils, salad dressings, and mayonnaise. They should be used only in moderation, and non-genetically modified and organic versions are the best choices. The healthiest polyunsaturated fats are found in walnuts, pumpkin seeds, sunflower seeds, and flaxseeds.

3. Monounsaturated Fats

These lower LDL cholesterol and are good for you. They can be found in avocados, olive oil, peanut oil, sesame oils, natural peanut butter, olives, sesame seeds, and most nuts.

4. Trans-fatty Acids

These are made when fats go through the chemical process of hydrogenation. This changes natural oils into semi-solid or solid fats. These are unnatural and harmful to your body. They are not metabolized in your body like natural fats and can result in a deformed cellular structure. You should carefully read labels and eliminate foods containing hydrogenated or partially-hydrogenated oils. Be careful—food manufacturers are allowed to label a product "contains 0% trans-fat" or "not a significant source of trans-fat" even if it contains equal or less than .5g per individual serving. Trans-fats are contained in many processed foods and mixes, breads, and fried and snack foods. Many companies have removed trans-fats from their products since the original labeling was created in 2006, so alternatives are easy to find.

5. **Essential Fatty Acids**

These are necessary fats that humans cannot make and must be obtained by diet. Some monounsaturated and polyunsaturated foods contain EFAs. There are two families: Omega-3 and Omega-6. Omega-9 is necessary yet "non-essential," because the body can manufacture a small amount on its own if 3 and 6 are present. EFAs support the cardiovascular, reproductive, immune, and nervous systems. They are needed to make and repair cell membranes, allowing the cells to obtain optimal nutrition and expel harmful waste. EFAs make prostaglandins which help to regulate body functions, such as heart rate, blood pressure, and blood clotting. They also help you to fight off infection and assist the immune system in regulating inflammation. They are needed for neural development and maturation of sensory systems in children, especially males.

Omega-3 deficiencies are linked to decreased mental abilities, tingling in the nerves, poor vision, a reduced immune system, learning disorders, and many other symptoms. Even though most Americans eat too much Omega-6, it is not always converted correctly in the body because of diets containing too much sugar, alcohol, and processed foods. Smoking, stress, aging, and viral infections can also reduce effectiveness. (I will cover which foods contain these EFAs in greater detail in upcoming chapters.)

WOW! I know that this chapter contains a lot of information to process and take in! I hope that it gave you a deeper understanding about how your body utilizes proteins, fats, carbohydrates, and water. I also hope that it increased your knowledge about how vitamins and minerals work synergistically to promote brain health and body healing. In the following chapters, I will show you what foods and substances hinder your ability to heal, what foods promote maximum energy and nutrition, where to find healthy options on the go, and wonderful, tasty recipes that are easy to make!

"Did you ever stop to taste a carrot? Not just eat it, but taste it? You can't taste the beauty and energy of the earth in a Twinkie." - Astrid Alauda

CHAPTER 3
What Foods to Avoid & Why

The food industry has a big problem, because they not only have to produce food, but they also have to distribute it to millions of people daily. This food has to be attractive and tasty enough to eat. This presents a conflict. Food that is fresh, has nutritional value, and is free of preservatives, like fresh fruit and vegetables, are fragile and expensive to deliver. Processed foods are cheap to produce, have a long shelf life, and are easy to store and distribute. Most foods that have a long shelf life have to be colorized to keep them looking fresh. They also have to be combined with various preservatives to stop them from degrading. This does not mean that you can never buy foods that are processed or convenient, but rather, you have to be diligent in reading the ingredients labels to fully understand what you are purchasing. The ingredient label is just as important, if not more so, than the level of calories, fat grams, etc. that is displayed above it. (I will be sharing with you healthy alternatives without the additives in upcoming chapters so that you have additional choices.)

There are certain things that you ingest, willingly and unknowingly, that directly affect the brain. Taking in neurotoxic substances is a form of malnutrition. These foods, additives, and preservatives can be toxic to brain cells, even in small amounts. The following topics will highlight how each affects your body and your brain.

Gluten and the Brain

Gluten sensitivity is now described as "one of the most common human diseases." There are about 3 million people currently in the US that are affected by this. Gluten sensitivity was originally seen to be only a gastrointestinal problem. However, recent research indicates that it can have a severe impact on the nervous system. Dr. Maios Hadjivassiliou of the United Kingdom, a recognized world authority on gluten sensitivity, indicates that people can have problems with brain function without any digestive issues at all.

Gluten is found in wheat, barley, kamut, rye, bulgur, and spelt. If you are gluten sensitive, your body produces elevated levels of antibodies against gliadin. These anti-gliadin antibodies turn on particular immune cells in your body. Then cytokines, which are inflammatory chemicals, are created. Cytokines are known to negatively affect brain function. In fact, elevated cytokines are seen in individuals with Alzheimer's disease, Parkinson's disease, multiple sclerosis, and autism. Because of the inflammation that this chemical reaction creates, brain function and ultimate brain health are compromised.

There is a lesser known condition called gluten ataxia. Although it belongs to the same group of gluten sensitivity as celiac disease, it is a disorder of the immune system. With this disorder, the focus of the disease is in the cerebellum of the brain. The cerebellum controls coordination, walking, speaking, and swallowing. Sometimes, the peripheral nerves coming off of the spinal cord are involved. These symptoms can appear as numbness, tingling, and pain, and they may progress into peripheral neuropathy.

Ataxia means loss of coordination. Neurological symptoms may appear as slurred speech, loss of coordination in limbs, difficulty walking, ocular problems, and recurrent headaches. In children and young adults, it can cause developmental delay, diminished muscle tone, and learning disorders.

According to Heidi Schwarz, M.D., a neurologist at the University of Rochester Medical Center and assistant professor of Neurology at Strong Memorial Hospital, "Gluten ataxia is out there, but so few of us have seen it—or perhaps recognized it. If you see a patient who has malabsorption problems, they can't tolerate this or can't tolerate that, if they have gastrointestinal complaints along with neurologic symptoms, then you order the antibody tests." Schwartz says, "Yet most patients I see with neurologic manifestations of gluten intolerance don't have a lot of GI symptoms, if any."

The blood test to screen for gluten ataxia is the same as the test to screen for gluten sensitivity. It measures the antigliadin antibodies (IgG and IgA) circulating in the blood.

Other neurological symptoms from sensitivity to gluten are the following:

- Headaches, migraines, or brain "fog"

- Joint and muscle pain

- Chronic fatigue and weakness

- Behavioral issues, seizures, depression, and psychiatric problems

If you are recovering from a Mild Traumatic Brain Injury, it is in your best interest to avoid products containing gluten, due to the neurological side effects, to optimize your recovery—even if you do not have the markers for gluten sensitivity or gluten ataxia. We are fortunate to live in a time where it is easy to avoid gluten and have many tasty, good quality options to choose from. (I promise!) I will reveal these to you in detail in future chapters.

If you are concerned that you may have food allergies and want to pursue getting Food Allergy & Food Sensitivity Testing done, I recommend a company that our Naturopath used, named BioTek. They were excellent. Not only did they provide us with results from each general category (like dairy), but they also broke the specifics down by each food (like cheddar cheese, cow's milk, mozzarella, etc.) There are many good Food Allergy & Food Sensitivity Labs in the US. We found that the blood testing done with this company through our Naturopath provided us with much more concrete information than a regular Allergist had done prior.

High Fructose Corn Syrup

High Fructose Corn Syrup was invented in Japan in 1966 and brought into the US in 1975. Food manufacturers started using it instead of sucrose (table sugar) because it costs three times less to make. High Fructose Corn Syrup began appearing in almost every pre-packaged and processed food on the market. In the past century, fructose consumption has increased by 5 times! The current intake of sugar per person is 141 pounds per year, 63 of which are from HFCS. Most adolescents are taking in 73 grams a day of fructose—12% of their daily caloric intake!

How does fructose affect your body? It interferes with the body's signals telling you that you are full. This happens because of a rise of leptin in your system, and it also does <u>NOT</u> stimulate ghrelin, which is the "hunger hormone." Because fructose raises insulin levels, it interferes with the communication between leptin and your hypothalamus; your brain senses that you are not satisfied by what you are eating and prompts you to eat more.

Because HFCS is man-made, it is converted into triglycerides and fat tissue, not usable blood glucose. HFCS is consumed in liquid form, usually in soda or as a food additive, so it affects your metabolism even faster.

Fructose contributes to the following:

- Insulin resistance and obesity
- Elevated blood pressure
- Higher triglycerides and LDL
- Cardiovascular disease, liver disease, arthritis, and gout

Fructose originates from fruits and vegetables. Past generations consumed about 15 grams a day compared to the 73 grams a day that the average adolescent consumes now. When you ingest fructose from foods, it's mixed with beneficial fiber, vitamins, phytonutrients, and enzymes—all of which balance out any negative metabolic effects. Fructose is not bad; it's the massive amount that the typical American consumes that has created the problems.

About ¼ of the calories consumed by the average American is in the form of added sugars. Believe it or not, the low-fat diet foods are the ones containing the most sugar. In most processed foods, all of the fiber has been removed, so there is barely any nutritional value left.

After ingesting fructose, 100% of the metabolic breakdown must happen in your liver. But with glucose, the liver only has to break down 20%. Every cell in your body, including your brain, uses glucose. So, much of it is used up very soon after it is ingested. However, fructose is turned into free fatty acids and gets stored as fat. These fatty acids accumulate in your liver and your skeletal muscle tissue, causing insulin resistance and non-alcoholic fatty liver disease. This metabolism by your liver creates an over abundance of uric acid in the body, which elevates blood pressure and may cause gout.

So, this is the straight scoop about high fructose corn syrup. Due to concerns about high fructose corn syrup and the health of the consumer, many food and beverage manufacturers are doing away with it. Knowledge is power, and you can decide how to become an advocate for your own health. I will discuss the healthiest sweeteners in the next chapter. Now let's take a look at those artificial sweeteners!

Artificial Sweeteners

People use artificial sweeteners because they are low in calories and are a sweet substitute for sugar. Aspartame is probably the most commonly one used, but how does it affect your brain? A study done by Humphries, Pretorius, and their colleagues from South Africa explains exactly that.

There are three components to aspartame: 50% phenylalanine, 40% aspartic acid, and 10% methanol. Phenylalanine is recognized as a neurotransmitter regulator. This study highlighted the possible negative effects on serotonin in the brain. Phenylalanine lowered the levels of serotonin, which then affected sleep, mood, appetite, and behavior. It also disrupted amino acid metabolism, hormone balance, and nerve functions. Aspartic acid works as an excitatory neurotransmitter in the central nervous system. Methanol is changed to formate, which is flushed out of the body or is accumulated in the body as formaldehyde.

Aspartame can also do the following:

- Disrupt protein metabolism

- Disrupt neuronal functions

- Cause improper functioning of enzymes

- Deplete the cells' ATP stores, which then lower the glucose levels, inhibiting the synthesis of acetylcholine and glutamate

Aspartame can cause an imbalance in brain chemicals, such as dopamine, norepinephrine, and epinephrine. These imbalances may manifest as headaches, insomnia, and seizures. This review-based study concluded that excessive intake of aspartame can lead to mental and emotional disturbances and may affect learning ability.

Currently, the following five artificial sweeteners are approved by the FDA:

1. **Aspartame**, sold under the brand names NutraSweet® and Equal®

2. **Saccharin**, sold under the brand name Sweet'N Low®

3. **Sucralose**, sold under the brand name Splenda®

4. **Acesulfame K** (or acesulfame potassium), produced by Hoechst, a German chemical company, widely used in foods, beverages, and pharmaceutical products around the world

5. **Neotame**, produced by the NutraSweet Company; the most recent addition to FDA's list of approved artificial sweeteners, used in diet soft drinks and low-calorie foods

The Center for Science in the Public Interest (CSPI) cautions everyone to avoid aspartame, saccharin, and acesulfame K, because they are unsafe in amounts consumed or are very poorly tested and not worth the risk.

Additional symptoms that have been associated with the consumption of aspartame include the following:

•	Nausea	•	Heart Arrhythmia
•	Dizziness	•	Hearing Loss
•	Tinnitus	•	Insomnia
•	Blurred Vision	•	Eye Problems
•	Hallucinations	•	Memory Loss
•	Personality Changes	•	Violent Episodes
•	Hyperactivity	•	Joint Pains
•	Numbness & Tingling	•	Fatigue
•	Mood Changes	•	Anxiety Attacks
•	Muscle Cramps	•	Skin Lesions

Fortunately, most of the above symptoms are alleviated once aspartame use is discontinued. Most individuals wouldn't even think to connect the above mentioned symptoms to artificial sweeteners.

Do you want to find out how sucralose (Splenda) negatively affects your health? A study done at Duke University determined that it reduces the healthy bacteria in your gut, which helps your immune system, by up to 50%. (Check out http://www.truthaboutsplenda. com.) Now you know!

Refined Sugar

Humans love sweet foods. We have been looking to satisfy our sweet tooth for centuries. Sugar is a simple carbohydrate that happens naturally in foods such as grains, beans, vegetables, and fruit. When it is left unprocessed, it is good for you.

Refined table sugar, which is sucrose, is very different. Derived from either sugar cane or beets, it lacks vitamins, minerals, and fiber, and it requires your body to work harder to digest it. Your body uses up its stored enzymes and minerals to absorb sucrose properly. What happens? Instead of your body receiving nutrition, it creates deficiency. It enters the blood stream rapidly affecting your body's blood sugar levels. When it is high, it causes excitability, nervous tension, and hyperactivity. When it drops low, it causes fatigue, exhaustion, and depression. Most people are aware that blood sugar levels fluctuate, but they do not recognize the emotional rollercoaster that comes along with it!

One of sugar's major drawbacks is that it raises your insulin level, inhibiting the release of hormones, which then reduces your immune system's ability to protect you against infection and disease. Back in 1970, Linus Pauling realized that white blood cells need a high dose of Vitamin C to fight the common cold. Because glucose and Vitamin C have similar chemical structures, they compete with each other to enter the cell. Too much sugar may reduce your white blood cells' ability to combat disease by up to 75%!

Sugar is actually considered to be an addictive substance because:

1. Eating even a small amount creates a desire for more; and

2. If you quit eating it suddenly, you may experience headaches, mood swings, cravings, and fatigue.

Where is sugar hidden in what we eat? How about canned vegetables, cereals, peanut butter, breads, and tomato sauce! Other names for refined sugar are corn syrup, dextrose, fructose, and maltose. Even some "healthy foods" contain sugar. A lemon poppy seed Cliff Bar has 21 grams of sugar, or 5 teaspoons. A chocolate glazed donut only has 14 grams comparatively! A 16 oz. Starbucks Frappuccino has 44 grams of sugar, or 10 teaspoons. This heavy intake of sugar has led to an explosion of hypoglycemia (blood sugar fluctuation) and Type II Diabetes.

How Sugar Affects Brain Health

According to Malcolm Peet, a noted British psychiatric researcher, there is a strong link between high sugar consumption and the risk of depression as well as schizophrenia. There are two ways that sugar may exert a toxic effect on mental health. First, BDNF, a key growth hormone in the brain, is suppressed by sugar. This hormone promotes the health of neurons in the brain and assists with memory by creating new neuron connections. Second, there is a cascade of chemical reactions that occur in the body when ingesting sugar that create chronic inflammation. Over time, inflammation suppresses the immune system, which then negatively affects brain function.

Dr. Ilardi, PhD, Associate Profession of Psychology at the University of Kansas, had some of his patients with depression give up simple sugars contained in crackers, white bread, and other refined foods. The patients that complied reported significant improvement in mood, energy, and mental clarity.

Because alcohol turns to sugar in the body, it should also be avoided. Alcohol can be a neurotoxin. According to the American Society for Nutrition, the single worst thing that you can do to your brain is to consume distilled spirits. Distilled spirits, such as vodka and rum, affect carbohydrates, which your brain needs to thrive, and they also slow down metabolism. Drinks also drain the body of Vitamin B and affect liver function.

After abstaining from sugar for months, my son decided over the Christmas break to eat sugar about five times in one day. That night he was lightheaded, dizzy, felt like "he was in a dream," and was anxious. He finally connected the two together, and he has decided not to repeat the experience!

As I mentioned earlier, I will share with you the healthiest sweeteners and also "sweet" foods that will enable you to transition to eating healthier and still be able to satisfy those sweet cravings. Want to check out a fun website to check how much sugar is contained in common foods? Go to http://sugarstacks.com/.

Partially Hydrogenated Oils

Partial hydrogenation is a chemical process that changes liquid oil into semi-solid or solid oil. Why? Because it provides a longer shelf-life for many processed foods, such as breads, mixes, stick margarine, icing, and fried and snack foods. They are also used as cooking oils for "frying" in restaurants.

Top nutritionists at Harvard have concluded that trans-fats may be responsible for as many as 30,000 premature coronary deaths a year. As mentioned in the "Nutrition and the Brain" chapter, they are not metabolized in your body like natural fats, and they can result in a deformed cellular structure. So what should you avoid?

- **Don't eat products with the words "shortening" or "partially hydrogenated" on the ingredients list**. NOTE: Fully hydrogenated oils (like beneficial coconut oil) <u>do not </u>contain trans-fats.

- **Even if the label says "no trans fat," be careful**. Food manufacturers are allowed to label a product "contains 0% trans-fat" or "not a significant source of trans fat" even if it contains equal or less than .5g per serving. Let's say that one serving contains .4g, but you eat 3 servings (which is totally possible). You've just taken in 1.2g of trans- fat, thinking that you are doing the right thing.

- **When dining out, don't be afraid to ask if they use trans-fats in their salad dressings, for frying, baking, etc**. When you ask, you are sending a message to the seller that you don't want trans-fats in your body.

You may have to search harder than you are accustomed to in avoiding partially hydrogenated oils. Many manufacturers have removed it from their products in the last couple of years. Be diligent. Once you find new products that you like, you can just grab it, because you will be past the learning curve. We'll get into healthier fat options in an upcoming chapter.

Artificial Food Dyes & Additives

Shopping was easy when all food came from farms. Now, factory-made foods have made chemical additives a significant part of our diet. Awareness is key, and knowledge allows you to make educated decisions for your own personal health. I am only going to highlight the worst dyes and additives to avoid, listed on the "Center for Science in the Public Interest" website. Don't worry. You'll be able to eat well without them!

- **Blue #2:** an artificial coloring in pet foods, candy, and beverages (like Gatorade!). Animal studies found some evidence that it causes brain cancer in male rats, even though the FDA concludes that "there is reasonable certainty of no harm."

- **Red #3:** Artificial coloring in candy and baked goods. According to a 1983 review report requested by the FDA, the fact that this dye caused thyroid tumors in rats was "convincing." However, it was never banned. It is still used in icing, gum, and fruit roll-ups.

- **Yellow #5:** Artificial coloring used in candy, pet foods, gelatin desserts, and baked goods. It is the second most common coloring used and can cause allergy-like hypersensitivity, primarily in people who are sensitive to aspirin. It can also cause hyperactivity in some children.

- **Yellow #6:** Artificial coloring in candy, baked goods, and beverages. Industry sponsored animal tests indicated that this dye, which is the third most commonly used, causes tumors of the adrenal glands and kidneys. It may cause hypersensitivity reactions in some individuals.

- **Butylated Hydroxyanisole (BHA):** An antioxidant in cereals, chewing gum, potato chips, and vegetable oil. BHA retards rancidity in fats, oils, and oil containing foods. The U.S. Department of Health & Human Services considers BHA to be "reasonably anticipated to be a human carcinogen." Nevertheless, the FDA still allows it to be used in our food.

- **Caramel Coloring:** Used primarily in colas. It's made by heating a variety of sugars with ammonium compounds or acids. By weight, it is the most widely used coloring added to foods and beverages. When caramel coloring is produced with ammonia, it produces a contaminant called 4-methylimidazole, which is also present in cigarette smoke. The amounts of this contaminant are so worrisome that the State of California has proposed that a warning notice be required on food and non-food products. It is worth avoiding colas and other beverages with this because the serving sizes are so large.

- **Monosodium Glutamate (MSG):** Used as a flavor enhancer in soups, salad dressing, chips, frozen entrees, and restaurant foods. This amino acid boosts the flavor in many foods. While this sounds great, it allows food manufacturers to reduce the amount of real ingredients in their foods, like chicken in chicken soup. As early as the 1960's, it was known that large amounts of MSG ingested by infant rats destroyed nerve cells in the brain. After this research was publicized, consumers forced baby food manufacturers to stop putting it in their products.

- **How can MSG affect the brain?** MSG may cross the blood-brain barrier and damage brain cells by excitatory neurotoxicity. Certain cells called oligodendrocytes, which are found in the nervous system and make myelin, are destroyed by excess glutamate. It is the inability to make myelin which defines the disease multiple sclerosis.

Other symptoms reported include: headaches, nausea, weakness, and a burning sensation on the back of the neck and forearms. Some people complain of wheezing, changes in heart rate, and difficulty breathing. People that are sensitive should be aware of other products containing glutamate. If you think that you have this sensitivity, here is a website for you: http://msgtruth.org.

- **Sodium Nitrites & Sodium Nitrates:** Used as a preservative and coloring in bacon, ham, deli meats, hot dogs, smoked fish, and corned beef. Meat processors love these additives, because they preserve the red coloring in meat (otherwise hot dogs and bacon would look grey). Several studies have linked consumption of cured meats and nitrite by children, pregnant women, and adults with various types of cancer. The meat industries justify using them by claiming it prevents the bacteria growth that cause botulism poisoning. This is true, but refrigeration and freezing prevent it as well. The use of nitrites and nitrates has been greatly reduced in the last decade. It is easy to find the above mentioned products without these ingredients at almost every market in the U.S.

- **Genetically Engineered & Genetically Modified Foods:** I'm sure that you have heard of (GE) and (GMO) foods. Most corn and soy seeds grown in the US have been genetically engineered so that they will be resistant to the pesticides that are sprayed on the plants to kill the insects. Yes, the plants thrive, but then these plants are harvested with pesticides like Roundup and put into our foods to be consumed. Do not purchase any soy products unless the label reads "Non-GMO."

Produce that is genetically modified will have a label marked by a 5 digit number beginning with an "8," like this: 84011. Buy conventional produce and wash with a veggie wash or buy organic produce instead.

Okay! That's it! I know that I have probably overwhelmed you with all of the seemingly negative information in this chapter! I did it for one reason only: so that you can be an informed advocate for your own health and to discover exactly what is in all of the above mentioned foods and additives that may hinder your state of well being and your recovery from Mild Traumatic Brain Injury.

I promise that the rest of this book will give you wonderful, tasty food options and recipes that are easy to find, easy to prepare and taste so good that you will forget all about what you cannot have! Be patient with yourself and take it one step at a time.

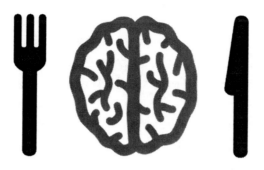

"You don't have to cook fancy or complicated masterpieces – just good food from fresh ingredients." – Julia Child

CHAPTER 4
Wonderful Foods That You Can Eat

Healthy eating is not about being perfect; it's about nourishing your body with the right foods for <u>you</u>. Many people think of the word "diet" as a rigid plan, but it doesn't have to be viewed that way! It simply requires a positive mindset shift to realize that the changes that you will make are for your benefit. It's important that you focus on the great healing foods that you can have instead of the foods that don't serve you well. Every time you eat and drink is a fresh opportunity to bring you back to being energetic and feeling better, and I am here to guide you along that path.

Eating well means consuming the foods that are the most "nutrient-dense." These are foods that are in their original form, like veggies and fruits, eggs, nuts, and animal products from animals in their natural environments. Some of these foods may look, smell, and taste different, especially if you have been indulging in a lot of processed foods. As with any important change, learning to eat better requires effort and persistence, but your brain will thank you for it!

Eating is very personal, and you may have emotional connections to certain foods or rituals. You don't have to deprive yourself or give up traditions; you just need to substitute them with healthier choices. In this book, I will show you tasty recipes, broken down by category, as well as "our favorites" for quick meals and on-the-go snacks, condiments, spices, etc. Good food does <u>NOT</u> have to be boring in flavor! I will also share with you websites of food manufactures that we love so that you won't feel overwhelmed with searching from scratch.

In this chapter, I will give you an overview of everything that you can eat with easy to use charts for quick reference. After you read it through, think about all of the ways that you can incorporate these foods into your diet. You won't like all of these items, but experiment. Listen to your body and eat the ones that work best for you and your lifestyle. Please be adventurous and eat "outside the box." You'll be sure to discover taste buds that you didn't even know you had!

Understanding the Glycemic Index

The Glycemic Index (GI) measures how quickly a food is digested and raises blood sugar levels. Carbohydrates are consumed, measured, and ranked according to their immediate effect on blood glucose (blood sugar) levels. Some researchers are now looking at the Glycemic Load (GL) to look at the full impact on your body's chemistry. It's calculated by multiplying the Glycemic Index by the amount of carbohydrates in the food. For example, a raw carrot has a high Glycemic Index of 131, but they contain only 4 grams of carbohydrates, for a low Glycemic Load of 5. It's all about bio-individuality. Try a food, see how you feel after eating it, and make your decision from there. If you would like more information regarding the Glycemic Index, there are many books and websites available to you.

Fruits & Vegetables

Fruits and vegetables are nutrient dense and low in calories, fat, and cholesterol, and they keep blood sugar levels stable. They contain vitamins, minerals, fiber, phytonutrients, and antioxidants that help to fight disease.

Good to Know

Pesticides on veggies and fruits kill weeds, fungus, and bugs. Conventional produce is sprayed heavily so that the plants/trees will have the highest yield possible. Waxes are applied to seal in moisture and extend the shelf life of the product. You want the nutrients but not the chemicals. It can be difficult because organic can be expensive and hard to find. However, buy organic when you can (frozen is fine). Next buy local and then conventional. (Do the best that you can—no punishment here!)

You can wash your produce in a couple of ways:

- Buy a vegetable and fruit wash, which is easy to find in the produce department of your grocery store. For more information, see: http://www.vegiwash.com/ or http://www.tryfit.com/; or

- Fill a clean spray bottle with equal parts white vinegar and filtered water. Spray it on your produce, rub it in, and rinse thoroughly. Soak thin-skinned produce for 5-10 minutes and rinse and dry thoroughly.

The Environmental Working Group's
Shopping Guide to Pesticides in Produce

Dirty Dozen	Clean Fifteen
Celery	Onions
Peaches	Avocado
Strawberries	Sweet Corn
Apples	Pineapple
Blueberries	Mangoes
Nectarines	Sweet Peas
Bell Peppers	Asparagus
Spinach	Kiwi
Cherries	Cabbage
Kale/Collard Greens	Eggplant
Potatoes	Cantaloupe
Grapes (imported)	Watermelon
	Grapefruit
	Sweet Potato
	Honeydew Melon

(You can even download an iPhone app of this list at their website: http://www.foodnews.org/.)

Reading Produce Labels

It's important to note that produce is labeled in the following way:

- "Conventionally Grown"   4 Digits - #4011

- "Organically Grown"   5 Digits - #94011

- "Genetically Modified"   5 Digits – (CAUTION!) #84011

When shopping for fruits and vegetables, as with any kind of food, pay attention to the labels, and know what you are putting into your body.

Good for You Fruits & Veggies

NOTE: There is a huge array of fruits and vegetables available in the world for you to try. Not all are listed here. The following charts provide you with an easy-to-use guide of the most common options. Whenever possible, limit or eliminate canned fruits in syrup (or rinse them thoroughly).

FRUITS

Fruit	The Good Stuff
Apple	Fiber and cholesterol-lowering pectin
Apricot	Protein, iron, calcium, zinc, Vitamin A, and beta carotene
Avocado	Good fat, fiber, and Vitamin E
Banana	Potassium
Blueberry	Vitamin C, manganese, and antioxidants
Cantaloupe	Vitamin C, beta carotene, and potassium
Cherry	Iron and beta carotene
Fig	Iron, calcium, fiber, and folic acid
Grapefruit	Low cal, fiber, and Vitamin C (Also try lemons & limes.)
Grape	Antioxidants, Vitamins A, B-complex, and C
Kiwi	Vitamin C, magnesium, and potassium
Mango	Vitamin A and C
Orange	Vitamin C, calcium, and pectin fiber (the white membrane has bioflavanoids) (Also try clementines and tangerines.)
Papaya	Vitamin A and C and the enzyme papain that aids digestion (Also try guava.)
Peach	Vitamin A and C and calcium (Also try nectarines.)
Pear	Pectin fiber, potassium, boron, and eases constipation
Pineapple	Manganese, Vitamin C, and digestive enzymes
Plum	Vitamin C (Also try dried—prunes.)
Pomegranate	Potassium and phytonutrients
Raspberry	Fiber, folic acid, zinc, and antioxidants (Also try blackberries.)
Strawberry	Vitamins A and C and fiber
Watermelon	Vitamins A and C and potassium

VEGETABLES

Vegetable	The Good Stuff
Asparagus	Vitamin A, B-complex, C and E, potassium, zinc, and glutathione
Artichoke	Potassium, iron, calcium, and magnesium
Beet	Magnesium, iron, and phosphorus (Try beet greens for salads.)
Broccoli	Vitamin C, calcium, and selenium
Cabbage	Vitamins C and E, calcium, chlorophyll, minerals, antioxidants, and phytonutrients
Carrot	Vitamin A and carotenoids (Also try parsnips.)
Celery	Vitamin A, B-complex, and C, choline, and potassium.
Cucumber	Silicon, water, and digestive enzymes
Eggplant	Potassium and water
Green Bean	Vitamin A and B-complex, calcium, and potassium
Kohlrabi	Vitamin C, potassium, and fiber
Leafy Greens	Vitamins A, C, E, and K, calcium, magnesium, fiber, zinc, iron, potassium, folic acid, and chlorophyll
Mushroom	Protein, Vitamin B, and zinc
Onion	Antibacterial, anticancer agents, and antioxidants (Also try leeks and garlic.)
Peppers	Vitamin C
Potato	Manganese, chromium, selenium, and molybdenum (Watch your intake, as it turns to sugar quickly.)
Pumpkin	Vitamin A, potassium, and helps regulate blood sugar
Squash	Vitamin A and C, potassium, and calcium
Sweet Potato	Vitamin A and C, calcium, and carotenoids (Also try yams.)
Tomato	Vitamin A, B, and C, potassium, and phytochemicals

FRUITS & VEGETABLES

Fruits	The Good Stuff
Berries	Vitamin C, pectin, and phytonutrients (Try blackberries, blueberries, raspberries, and strawberries.)
Citrus	Vitamin C and potassium. (Try clementines, grapefruit, lemon, lime, oranges, and tangerines.)
Melons	Beta-carotene and potassium (Try canary, cantaloupe, casaba, Crenshaw, honeydew, and watermelon.)
Vegetables	**The Good Stuff**
Cruciferous	Calcium, magnesium, iron, Vitamins A and C, anti-cancerous, and phytonutrients (Try arugula, beet greens, bok choy, broccoli, brussels sprouts, cabbage, cauliflower, chard, collards, daikon, endive, kale, kohlrabi, mustard greens (strong), and watercress.)
Roots/Tubers	Fiber, potassium, beta-carotene, and Vitamin C (Try beets, burdock, carrots, celery root, daikon, onion, parsnip, potato, radish, rutabaga, sweet potato, turnip, and yam.)
Squash (summer)	Vitamins A and C, potassium, and calcium Try pattypan, scallop, yellow, and zucchini.
Squash (winter)	Vitamins A and C, potassium, iron, riboflavin, and magnesium (Try acorn, butternut, chayote, pumpkin, and spaghetti.)

✖ Gluten-Free Whole Grains

In their natural state, gluten-free whole grains contain complex carbs, proteins, fiber, unsaturated fats, B vitamins, Vitamin E, iron, zinc, and magnesium. They can be soaked, sprouted, cooked whole, rolled, flaked, or ground into flours.

<u>Good to Know:</u>

Don't eat too many refined grains with additives that you don't need. Grains have three layers: the germ, the bran, and the endosperm. When they are refined, the high-fiber, outer layer of bran and the germ (which is nutrient dense) are removed. The endosperm that remains is ground and processed with bleaching agents. Then synthetic vitamins are added and the product is labeled "enriched" or "fortified."

Eating products that are refined, like white rice, white bread, and refined flour, causes your body to pull the missing nutrients in these foods from your bones, tissues, and other reserves to metabolize and digest these foods. Because they lack fiber, they are digested quickly and cause a rise in blood sugar, insulin, and energy. Thus explains the blood sugar rollercoaster. So make sure that you choose to eat from the following list of gluten-free whole grains:

WHOLE GRAINS (GLUTEN-FREE)

Whole Grain	The Good Stuff
Amaranth (Use with cereals or mix with other grains.)	Protein, calcium, and iron
Brown Rice (Use in everything-even for breakfast.)	Available in short, medium or long grains. Contains fiber, protein, and Vitamin E.
Buckwheat (Known as Kasha – Gluten-Free) (Use in salads and pilafs.)	Contains thiamin, riboflavin, calcium and phosphorus.
Millet (Use in hot cereals, puddings and soups.)	Tiny gold seed. Contains thiamin, iron, protein and potassium. It is easily digested.
Oats (look for Gluten-Free versions) (Use in cereals or use whole oats in soups & salads.)	Available whole, steel-cut, rolled or quick-cooking. Contains fiber, protein, and B vitamins.
Quinoa (Use in salads or pilafs or for breakfast.)	Small, pearly grain loaded with protein. Contains calcium, iron, phosphorus, and B-vitamins.
Wild Rice (Use in salads and pilafs and casseroles.)	Contains protein, choline, folate, magnesium, phosphate and potassium.

Fish

Fish are an excellent source of protein and minerals, such as magnesium, zinc, phosphorus, omega- 3's, and iron. They are low in saturated fat and easy for the body to digest.

Good to Know:

Fish include freshwater, saltwater, and shellfish. We have increased our fish consumption over 200% since the 1960's. This has created concerns such as over-fishing, contamination, and issues around fish-farming (aquaculture). Both farmed and wild fish can become contaminated from polluted waters or if they are improperly handled. So, how can you make the best choices for you? There is a wonderful organization called the Blue Ocean Institute that has created a great guide. Below I've highlighted some of the best known choices. Please go to their website for more detailed information (www.blueocean.org).

Check This Out:

Go to their site: http://www.blueocean.org/home, and you can download their "Fish Phone." This allows you to know immediately if the fish you want to buy is safe and sustainable. How's that for immediate gratification?

**Abundant Species
Fishing/Farming Methods Cause
Little Damage to the Environment**

- Albacore Tuna, U.S. pole and troll caught
- Atlantic Mackerel
- Bay Scallops, farmed
- Eastern Oyster, farmed
- Crawfish, U.S. farmed
- Alaskan Salmon
- Sardines
- Striped Bass
- Yellow Fin Tuna, pole and troll caught

**Medium to High Abundance
Fishing/Farming Methods Cause
Some Damage to the Environment**

- Albacore Tuna, imported
- American Lobster
- Catfish, U.S. farmed
- Bluefish
- Pacific Cod
- Pacific Halibut
- Shrimp, U.S. farmed
- Swordfish, Atlantic and Mediterranean

Some Problems Exist with Fishing/Farming Methods Information is Insufficient for Evaluation
• Blue Crab
• Monkfish
• Catfish, farmed and imported
• Salmon, California, Oregon & Washington
• Sea Scallops
• Shrimp, Southeastern U.S.
• Swordfish, Pacific Ocean

Abundance is Low, and Product Is Overfished Serious Environmental Impact
• Albacore Tuna, longline caught
• Skate
• Tilapia, Central & South America farmed
• Atlantic Bluefin Tuna
• Atlantic Cod, U.S. & Canada
• Atlantic Salmon, farmed
• Chilean Sea Bass
• Shark, imported

⊠ Meats

Meat includes beef, pork, lamb, and "game" meats, such as bison, deer, rabbit, and buffalo. It's a good source of protein, iron, zinc, selenium, phosphorus, and B vitamins. Pasture raised and grass-fed animals contain less fat, more Vitamin E and greater amounts of conjugated linoleic acid (CLA)—an important essential fatty acid.

Good to Know:

Today, most animals that are raised for consumption are transferred to overcrowded feedlots where they are bred, not fed their natural diet, injected with hormones, and treated with low level antibiotics for the sole purpose of getting them to market as quickly as possible. These conditions can lead to unhealthy animals, which, in turn, can lead to unhealthy people.

Meat has been nourishing cultures for thousands of years before the rise of heart disease and high cholesterol. The animals were allowed to roam and eat grass, and they were not fed grains that now cause the meat to contain high levels of saturated fats. If you choose to eat grain-fed meats, trim off all of the excess fat, eat smaller portions, and limit how often you eat it.

As mentioned in the last chapter, prepared meats, such as bacon, lunch meats, sausages, and hot dogs, contain toxic additives, such as BHA, BHT, and sodium nitrate. When cooked at high temperatures, sodium nitrate turns into nitrosamine, which is a potent carcinogenic compound that your brain and your body do NOT need! Look for healthier versions of these products without these nitrates.

Search for products that are hormone-free and antibiotic-free, are raised in humane conditions, and are processed properly. (Most supermarkets carry at least some of the above; if not, ask them to!) You can Google "local farmers" in your area for the best quality and to support your local businesses. (Sources are provided for you in the "Resources" chapter of this book.) Most community farms offer produce, dairy, and meat.

MEATS

Feed Yourself Well With
- Meats that are free of antibiotics and hormones that are safely handled and safely processed; and/or
- Organic and/or pasture-fed animals.

Meats	The Good Stuff
Beef Chuck Rib Loin Flank Sirloin Round	Graded by Prime, Choice, Select; cubes, strips, tips neck, shoulder, blade rib or rib-eye shell, tenderloin under the loin behind flank, loin ground meat
Pork Shoulder Loin Belly Leg	 rump, picnic shoulder pork chops, tenderloins ribs, bacon ham
Lamb	legs, chops, rack, loin, shoulder, shank, breast
Cured-meats	ham, bacon, lunch meats, and sausages

✖ Poultry & Eggs

Poultry and eggs are wonderful sources of protein for a healthy brain. Poultry that is allowed to roam in the pasture contain high levels of Omega-3's, Vitamins A and E, folic acid, and carotenoids. Eggs are affordable and easy to prepare, and they contain choline, Vitamins A, B2 and B12, selenium, iron, folate, and other trace nutrients.

Good to Know:

Chickens can be raised either free-range (allowed to roam), cage-free (housed, but un-caged), or factory farmed. Without getting into the gruesome details of factory farming, these birds are not the most nutrient dense. They are put on antibiotics to minimize disease (which we then ingest), and they are bred to grow as large as possible in the shortest amount of time. Cage-free birds are housed in environments with room to express their natural behaviors, and they are usually fed a quality vegetarian diet, supplemented with Omega-3 fatty acids. If they are labeled "naturally raised," their beaks are not clipped, and antibiotics are not used. Free-range birds are free to roam in fenced areas, and they have access to grasses, which increase their nutritional quality.

Eggs have cholesterol in the yolk; however, research now shows that there is little correlation between dietary cholesterol and blood cholesterol levels. Individuals with high cholesterol, diabetes, or heart disease may want to limit their consumption of egg yolks. Others are safe to eat 1-2 eggs daily. The most nutrient dense eggs are from free-range hens or cage-free birds fed diets that are supplemented with flax or fish meal. You can usually find all of the above products in your neighborhood markets. In our city supermarkets, I am able to purchase excellent quality, local eggs affordably.

POULTRY AND EGGS

Feed Yourself Well With
- Cage-free poultry and eggs, enhanced with Omega-3 fatty acids; and/or
- Free-range or pastured poultry and eggs.

Poultry	The Good Stuff
Birds Chicken Duck Goose Turkey	May be cooked whole, in parts or ground. Can be roasted, baked, grilled, broiled, sautéed, or stir-fried. Ground can be used in meatloaf, chili, burgers, and other dishes.
Bird Products Sausages Hot dogs Deli meats	Purchase only products with no MSG, nitrates, artificial colors or flavors. Use sausages in soups, casseroles, stews, etc.
Game Birds Guinea hen Partridge Pheasant & Quail	Usually farm raised. Pheasant may be domestic or wild (stronger flavor). Quail is sweet and tender.
Eggs	Hens fed a healthy diet with flax or fish meal to increase Omega-3 fatty acids, from cage-free, free-range, or pastured poultry

✠ Dairy

Butter, milk, cream, cheese, and yogurt come primarily from cows, but they can also come from sheep and goats. Dairy products contain amounts of protein, fats, carbohydrates, calcium, Vitamins A, B2, and other B vitamins, phosphorus, magnesium, potassium, and sodium. Grass-fed cows yield much more nutrient dense by-products.

Good to Know:

Dairy is a prominent industry in our current society, yet there is much confusion surrounding its consumption. Our society emphasizes that dairy is a very important source of calcium. However, cultures with little or no dairy intake have the strongest teeth and bones. Some Asian cultures ingest less than half of the recommended daily allowance for calcium, yet they have the lowest rates of osteoporosis and bone fractures. In our country, 25% of our diet is from dairy, yet we have the highest number of fractures and osteoporosis. Many cultures with strong bones may consume calcium in forms that are more readily absorbed by the body, eat more alkaline-forming foods (like vegetables), get more exercise, and consume fewer calcium inhibiting items like soda and sugar.

Milk is usually processed in the following three ways:

- **Pasteurized:** heated to destroy harmful bacteria and enzymes that sour the milk.

- **Homogenized:** breaks up fat globules to provide a uniform consistency so cream doesn't rise.

- **Fortified:** provides synthetic vitamins, like A and D, to help with calcium absorption.

Many people in the nutritional field would like to see the return of raw milk products. They state that past sanitary concerns that lead to the need for pasteurization are no longer relevant and that certified raw milk from healthy, pasture-fed cows is the least processed and most nutritious.

Pasteurization can destroy or denature enzymes and beneficial bacteria that help to break down lactose (milk sugar) and casein (milk protein), which can cause health issues. This is why raw, fermented, and "cultured" dairy items, such as yogurt, cheeses, buttermilk, and cottage cheese, are easier to digest and absorb. This, however, is an individual decision for you to make.

NOTE: Some states allow raw milk products to be sold commercially; in others, they must be bought directly from a local farm. Many health authorities oppose the consumption of unpasteurized milk, and it is forbidden to transport raw milk across state lines.

Want more information? Check out this site: http://www.raw-milk-facts.com/.

Casein, the protein in milk, can be very difficult to digest, and it is a very common food allergy. Many people do not understand that physical ailments, such as cramping, bloating, diarrhea, ear infections, sinus problems, and eczema, may be connected to their intake of dairy products. If you are concerned, eliminate dairy products for 1-2 weeks and see if your symptoms improve.

Now, let's discuss the issue of "obtaining calcium." Taking in calcium is different from absorbing and utilizing calcium. In order for it to be used by the body properly, calcium requires the proper balance of other nutrients, especially magnesium. Because many people eat a diet that is high in acid-producing foods (like coffee, soda, animal proteins, and refined flour products), the acid/alkaline balance that is <u>SO</u> important for the body's internal environment is altered. Because your body is always trying to maintain balance, it will leach calcium and other alkalinizing minerals from your bones to neutralize the acid. This can lead to depletion of calcium reserves and the thinning of bones.

Magnesium plays a huge role in the absorption and proper use of calcium as well as other nutrients. As a matter of fact, magnesium is responsible for over 300 chemical reactions required for your body's optimum health. Dairy products are high in calcium but low in magnesium. Whole grains, leafy green vegetables, and beans contain calcium and magnesium, along with other nutrients which help to move calcium into the bones. In a nutshell, you need calcium, AND you need foods containing magnesium to metabolize it correctly.

What About Butter?

Butter is made from the cream of churned milk. It contains Vitamins A, D, K, and E and essential fatty acids as well as selenium, an antioxidant. Your body uses these natural fats for energy. Many people avoid using butter because it is high in saturated fats and cholesterol. However, did you know that butter contains lecithin which helps to break down and metabolize cholesterol? Butter is a whole food that is a better nutrition choice than shortening or margarines that contain trans-fatty acids. (A side note, since my younger son has been consuming small amounts of butter, his eczema has disappeared!)

DAIRY

What to Limit or Eliminate:
- Dairy products that contain bovine growth hormones (BGH) and antibiotics;
- Dairy with artificial additives, sweeteners, and colorings; and
- Margarines and vegetable shortening.

Feed Yourself Well With:
- Dairy free of hormones or organic; and or
- Fermented or cultured dairy.

Dairy	The Good Stuff
Butter	Churned cream. Can use clarified butter (ghee) which is free of lactose and casein.
Cheese Hard Semifirm Soft Semisoft	Protein, calcium, phosphorus, vitamin A, fat and sodium. Parmesan, Romano Cheddar, Swiss Brie, Camembert Havarti, Provolone
Cottage cheese	Cultured mixed with cream and salt
Cream	Fat from whole milk, can be light or heavy, ½ and ½ is a mixture of milk and cream, also sour cream (cultured)
Cream cheese	Cultured cream, high in fat and cholesterol

Milk	Skim, low-fat, whole, flavored,
Certified Raw	Available in some states
Goat	Structure different than cow; easily digested
Buttermilk	Cultured or "soured"; easily digested
Yogurt	Fermented milk, look for "active yogurt cultures", Greek (more protein), Kefir – milk-based drink

HIGH CALCIUM FOODS

- Hard cheeses (like Parmesan)
- Dried seaweed (hijiki, wakame, kelp, Kombu). This may be new to you. However, people use them all the time. An easy way to incorporate it is to put a small piece into your stews/soups. The vitamins will leach out, and there is no detectable flavor. Remove the piece before serving.)
- Sardines
- Almonds
- Amaranth (grain)
- Greens (collard, kale, turnip, etc.)
- Quinoa (grain)
- Tofu (buy only non-GMO versions)
- Milk (buy only organic or no rGBH)
- Beans (black, pinto, garbanzo – rinse thoroughly)
- Yogurt
- Seeds (sunflower, sesame)
- Nuts (Brazil, walnuts)
- Figs
- Salmon

HIGH MAGNESIUM FOODS
• Dried seaweed • Beans (soy, mung, aduki,, black – buy only non-GMO soy beans) • Buckwheat • Millet • Nuts (almonds, cashews, filberts) • Seeds (sesame) • High-chlorophyll foods (green plants, microalgae, such as spirulina and chlorella)

✠ Legumes (Beans)

Legumes are chock full of nutrients and contain protein, complex carbohydrates, soluble and insoluble fiber, potassium, calcium, iron, zinc, folic acid, B vitamins, and phytonutrients. They are low in fat, can be easily found, and are not expensive. They can be purchased either dried or canned. (When using canned beans, rinse them thoroughly.)

Good to Know:

Legumes are a great natural whole food, and they are a good protein option instead of meat. Because they contain complex sugars, they can be difficult to digest for some. When these sugars are broken down in the intestines by bacterial enzymes, they can cause gas and abdominal discomfort. Ingesting a couple drops of liquid Beano or soaking dried beans prior to cooking can help. (Soaking beans helps to neutralize phytic acid which can interfere with mineral absorption.) Don't let this possible side effect stop you!! There is great flexibility in incorporating beans into your diet—sprinkle them on a salad, make chili, make a bean dip, or add them to a hearty soup.

Be careful when consuming soybeans. Our society's food manufacturers use soy as an inexpensive ingredient in prepared and packaged foods. They are cheap, easy to grow, are a high-pesticide crop, and are usually genetically engineered. What does that mean to you? Pesticide manufactures have genetically engineered soybeans to be resistant to the many pesticides that are sprayed on them (like Monsanto's Roundup). The beans survive to be harvested, but you are consuming the pesticides along with the product. Purchase only non-GMO or organic soy products.

In 30 countries around the world, including Australia, Japan, and all of the countries in the European Union, there are significant restrictions or outright bans on the production of GMO's, because they are not proven safe.

Want to learn more? Check out: http://www.nongmoproject.org/consumers/about-gmos/

How do you cook dried beans? Discard cracked or shriveled beans and any that look nasty. Place dried beans in water 3-4 times their volume for 8 hours or overnight. Throw away the soaking liquid and add fresh water 2 inches above the beans. Boil for 10 minutes and then cover, simmering until tender. That's it!

LEGUMES (Beans)

Feed Yourself Well With:
- Dried beans; and
- Rinsed canned beans.

Legume	The Good Stuff
Adzuki	Small, dark, red, calcium, iron, potassium and Vitamin A
Black Beans (turtle)	Strong flavor, good for soups and "refried"
Black-eyed Pea	Have a notable black spot; cook quickly
Garbanzo (chickpea)	Potassium, calcium, iron, and Vitamin A
Kidney	Red or white (cannellini)
Lentils	Brown, green and red varieties. No soaking needed. Potassium, protein, calcium, magnesium, phosphorus and sulfur
Lima	Potassium, phosphorus and Vitamin A
Mung	Green, common in Asia. Digested easily
Peas	Calcium, potassium, and phosphorus. Snow and sugar snap. Can be used in a variety of dishes
Pinto	Vitamins A and B, calcium, potassium
Split Peas	Green or yellow. No soaking needed
White	Navy and great northern
Soybean (Use only non-GMO)	Complete protein, iron, isoflavones, B vitamins. Edamame (green , immature)

✷ Healthy Fats (Nuts & Seeds)

Nuts and seeds are really nutritious because they are whole foods that contain good fats, protein, essential fatty acids (EFA's), fiber, B vitamins, folic acid, calcium, potassium, magnesium, iron, zinc, Vitamin E, and selenium.

Good to Know:

Nuts and seeds in their whole form are not only nutritious but shelf stable. Chopped nuts and seeds spoil quickly. You can store them in sealed containers in the refrigerator for up to three months. You can use them for snacks, trail mix, salads, breads, cookies, casseroles, or you name it! Nuts and seeds can also be ground into tasty butters. Do **NOT** buy any nut butters that contain added sugars or hydrogenated oils. If your peanut butter has oil floating on top, (which is a good thing), either store it upside down, or after opening, use a bread knife to blend. Be adventurous and try cashew butter, almond butter, sunflower seed butter, etc.

- Almond butter is great for dips and spreads, and it contains 8 times more calcium than peanut butter and 4 times more calcium than milk! (We drink unsweetened vanilla almond milk daily and use it for smoothies, drinking, mashed potatoes, etc. It's our favorite, and it tastes good!)

- Cashew butter is heartier, and it is good for spreading on bread and thickening smoothies and soups.

- Sesame seed butter (tahini) and hummus (from chickpeas and tahini) are good spreads.

NUTS AND SEEDS

What to Eliminate:
- Conventional nut butters containing hydrogenated oils, sugar, or other additives

Feed Yourself Well With:
- Fresh, whole nuts and seeds (organic if you can)
- Nut and seed butters: almond, cashew, macadamia, sunflower, and sesame.

Nuts	The Good Stuff
Almond	Potassium, magnesium, and calcium
Brazil Nut	Potassium, phosphorus, calcium, and sulfur
Cashew	Magnesium, phosphorous, potassium, and Vitamin A
Chestnut	Higher carbs and lower fat than most nuts
Coconut	Technically a fruit; try dry or flaked and coconut milk
Filbert	(Hazelnut) Potassium, phosphorus, calcium, and sulfur
Macadamia	Sweet – 70% fat
Peanut	Technically a legume; protein, fat, B vitamins & iron
Pecan	Phosphorus, potassium, amd Vitamin A
Pine Nut	(Pignolia) Fat , vitamins and minerals
Pistachio	Protein, calcium, Vitamin A, iron, and potassium
Walnut	Omega-3's, calcium, magnesium, potassium, Vitamin A, and zinc

Seeds	The Good Stuff
Alfalfa	(Can buy as sprouts) Vitamins A, D, E, and K
Flax	Omega-3's; healthy, can aid digestion and may have a laxative effect
Pumpkin	Iron, phosphorus, Vitamin A & zinc
Sesame	Calcium, potassium, phosphorus, magnesium, and Vitamin A
Sunflower	Potassium, phosphorus, silicon, calcium, and Vitamin A

❖ Healthy Oils

Oils come from nuts and legumes, fruits (avocados and olives), and fish. These oils improve brain function, give you energy, help your body use vitamins, build healthy cells, create healthy skin and hair, make hormones, cushion your organs, and help you to feel full and satisfied.

Good to Know:

There are three types of fats: saturated, monounsaturated, and polyunsaturated. The difference in their "saturation" determines the solidity of the fat at room temperature. The more saturated fats, like butter and coconut oil, are solid at room temperature. These are the most stable fats because they are able to resist damage from heat and oxidation, and they are best for high-temperature cooking and baking. In a moment, I will get into the GREAT benefits of coconut oil for your brain and your body.

Monounsaturated oils, like olive oil and sunflower oil, can withstand moderate heat and can be used for low-temperature cooking. Expeller pressed, extra-virgin olive oil is the most desirable, and it can be used in salad dressings, marinades, etc. Try to purchase it in a dark bottle as this increases its shelf life.

Polyunsaturated fats, found in walnuts, safflower, and flax oils, are very delicate and should not be exposed to heat, light, or oxygen. These oils should be uses as marinades and dressings and as a flavoring on top of cooked vegetables or grains. Flax seed is an amazing source of Omega-3 fatty acid. You can use ground flax seeds in yogurt, smoothies, salads, baking, and more! Purchase flax seed oil in a dark bottle and store it in the refrigerator. Do not use for cooking.

Avocados are a very healthy fat, and they are considered a fruit because they contain a seed. Each serving of an avocado (one fifth of a whole avocado) contains over 20 vitamins, minerals, and phytonutrients. How can they help to heal your brain? They specifically contain Vitamin E for tissue repair and B6 and niacin for the nervous system and oxygen transport, magnesium for muscle and nerve function, and zinc for wound healing. Plus, they taste great!

Coconut oil is re-emerging as one of the healthiest oils for your body. I say "re-emerging," because before the campaigns in the 1950's to ban saturated fats, it was widely used as a healthy tropical oil. As a matter of fact, cookbooks as far back as the 19th century recommended it. Not all saturated fats are the same because some saturated fats occur naturally, while others are artificially manipulated using hydrogenation (see partially hydrogenated oils in the previous chapter).

I bet that you didn't know that people in many tropical Pacific island locations that get between 30-60% of their caloric intake from coconut oil have hardly any cardiovascular disease! If fact, coconut oil contains amazing natural properties that are great for your body and your overall health. Why? Coconut oil contains a fat called lauric acid that your body converts into monolaurin. Monolaurin has anti-bacterial, anti-viral, and anti-protozoa properties. Coconut oil is known to contain more lauric acid than any other product on Earth.

Coconut oil is made up of about 2/3 medium–chain fatty acids (MCFA's). These fatty acids have been shown to produce the following health benefits:

- Promote heart health

- Promote weight loss (a side note: in the 1940's farmers tried to fatten up their cows by giving them coconut oil and found that they became strong and lean instead!)

- Support the immune system

- Support a healthy metabolism

- Provide you with an immediate energy source (great for athletes!)

- Keep your skin and hair beautiful

- Support the proper functioning of your thyroid gland

These fats in coconut oil are so nutritious that they have been used in infant formula, for helping people with digestive problems, and in hospitals to feed the critically ill.

So how can coconut oil help your brain? A study reported in the European Journal of Internal Medicine took a scientific look at the connection between nutrition and Alzheimer's disease. In layman's terms, they concluded that the early causes of Alzheimer's centered around the transport of cholesterol from the blood stream to the brain.

The brain is highly dependent on cholesterol. Even though the brain represents only 2% of the body's mass, it utilizes 25% of the body's cholesterol. Cholesterol is needed in the brain as an antioxidant, as an electrical insulator (to prevent ion leakage), to support the neural network, and for all membranes to function properly. Cholesterol is also used to wrap and deliver neurotransmitters and plays an important part in the formation of synapses. A diet that contains the right amount of healthy saturated fats is essential to maintaining these cholesterol levels in individuals that have deficiencies in, or are suffering from, neurological disorders.

So, there you have it! Why WOULDN'T you make sure you ingested some healthy coconut oil daily? It's now readily available in your local market and also online. (Virgin Organic is best.) It's great to cook with, bake with, etc. It has an extremely long shelf life, and it does not go rancid for up to 2 years. If you live in an area above 76 degrees, coconut oil will be in liquid form; below 76 degrees, it is a solid until you cook with it. It can sustain high temperature cooking, and it is a very clean oil. It has no smell. (No, it does not smell like suntan lotion!)

PLANT OILS

What to Eliminate:
- Hydrogenated oils
- Trans-fatty acids
- Overly refined oils
- Oxidized oils (rancid after exposure to light and oxygen)

Feed Yourself Well With:
- Expeller-pressed
- Unrefined plant oils

Oil	The Good Stuff
Canola	High pesticide crop, buy organic; use in baking and medium-heat cooking
Coconut	Tropical oil, buy unrefined, very stable, very healthy; use for baking, high-heat cooking, in smoothies, etc.
Flax	High in Omega3's; refrigerate, use on salads, veggies, grains, in smoothies, etc. Do not cook with it – breaks down in heat.
Grapeseed	Can be used in medium-high heat cooking
Olive	Great flavor, stable, long shelf life (in dark bottle), use extra virgin; low-heat cooking
Palm	Tropical, stable oil, buy unrefined, use in high-heat cooking
Peanut	Stable, (try to find organic b/c of pesticide use); medium-high heat cooking
Safflower	Buy unrefined; use as dressing and for low-heat cooking
Sesame	Good flavor, (can buy toasted for stronger flavor),stable, long shelf life; medium-heat cooking

| Sunflower | Buy expeller pressed, use on salads, grains, veggies; not for cooking |
| Walnut | Buy expeller pressed, use on salads, grains, veggies; not for cooking |

⊞ Healthy Sweeteners

The best way to use natural sweeteners is to eat them the way nature intended—with all their nutrients intact. Eat wholesome, unrefined sweeteners combined with other nutrient-dense foods in moderation. Choose natural sweeteners that concentrate nutrients through boiling, reducing, and evaporation, like molasses, grain syrups, and jams. Blackstrap molasses contains chromium, calcium, and iron, and dark honey contains high levels of antioxidants. Even so, when recovering from a Traumatic Brain Injury, ALL sugars should be the LAST ingredient on your list to take in.

Good to Know:

As I mentioned earlier, the average American ingests over 150 pounds of sugar every year! As a result, most people are experiencing the blood sugar rollercoaster side effects and ill health. When your blood sugar is high, it can create excitability, nervous tension, and feelings of uneasiness. When it is low, it causes fatigue, exhaustion, and depression.

When you are recovering from a Mild Traumatic Brain Injury, you cannot afford to have anything that is in your control get in the way of your healing. Remember, I stated in the previous chapter that when you eat a lot of sugar, you are reducing your immune system's ability to protect you by up to 75%! Also, the hormone that creates healthy neurons and assists with memory is compromised by sugar intake. Most importantly, the chronic inflammation that occurs further suppresses the immune system and negatively affects brain health.

However, most of us have a sweet tooth, right? The best choices are to stock your pantry with fresh fruit, jellies, and jams with no added sugar and to use small amounts of sweeteners that will not elevate your blood sugar very much. When you eat fruit, the fiber slows down the uptake of sugars into the blood stream and makes you feel full. If you substitute nut butters for sweeteners, the fat in the butter accomplishes the same. Raid your spice cabinet (if you have one), and use cinnamon, nutmeg, and pure vanilla to sweeten things up.

Some people find transitioning to "sweet foods" very helpful. Some of these are sweet potatoes, carrots, yams, beets, and even onions (which are very sweet when caramelized in a pan!) Because these foods are "root vegetables," they are energetically grounding as well.

Okay, so sweet veggies are not good enough for you? Well, dark chocolate rules! Dark chocolate contains antioxidant compounds that are rich with flavonoids, phenols, and magnesium. Make sure you read the labels well and buy good quality chocolate with chocolate liquor and cocoa with no hydrogenated oils and excess sugar. Over 60% + is best. My son eats 2 pieces of 72% chocolate every day, and he loves it!

SWEETENERS

What to Limit or Eliminate:
- Regular sugar
- Brown sugar
- Fructose
- Corn syrup
- Artificial sweeteners

Feed Yourself Well With:
- Naturally sweet foods like fruit and sweet veggies
- Dark chocolate
- Less-refined sugars.

Sweetener	The Good Stuff
Agave Nectar	Low glycemic sweetener from the Blue Agave cactus; must be highly processed to achieve consistency, 1.4 times sweeter than sugar; if used for baking, reduce oven temperature by 25 degrees
Barley Malt	Naturally present enzymes, can be in powder or liquid form, strong flavor like molasses
Brown Rice Syrup	Tastes like moderately sweet butterscotch; ¼ cup = 1 c. reg. sugar; not great for diabetics because it contains some glucose
Date Sugar	Finely ground, dehydrated dates, utilizing this fruit's vitamin, mineral & fiber content. Can be used as a topping, in baking & in hot or cold cereals
Fruit Products	Jams, jellies, spreads; use organic if possible. Can use in baking

Dark Honey	Has natural enzymes, sweeter than sugar; use minimally.
Maple Syrup	Only buy REAL maple syrup; grade B has more minerals and is less refined. Use minimally as it elevates blood sugar (We use an Agave & Maple Syrup blend from Trader Joe's)
Molasses	Organic molasses is very nutritious and is made by clarifying and blending the extracted juices; iron, calcium, & magnesium
Rapadura	Organic, rich in vitamins and unrefined; ground, fine texture
Stevia	Leafy herb used for centuries by native South Americans; does not elevate blood sugar; 100 times sweeter than sugar; white is more refined; has zero calories. Use in drinks, baking, and cooking
Sucanat	Sugar Cane Natural; powder. Refined mechanically instead of through a chemical process so it retains its vitamins & minerals
Sugar Alcohols	Mannitol, sorbitol, xylitol; sugar substitutes. OK for diabetics because it does not elevate blood sugar, may cause intestinal issues
Vegetable Glycerin	Colorless, odorless liquid syrup; sweet taste. Derived from coconut and palm oils. Good for people with candida because it does not contain sucrose

| Palm Sugar | Extracted from the sago and coconut palm trees; low glycemic; widely used throughout Southeast Asia; varied color from light to dark brown; minimally processed; molasses like flavor |
| Yacon Syrup | Freshly pressed from the Yacon root in the Andes; glucose free; contains medicinal properties to assist immune system in fighting bacteria; sweet taste; rich in iron, calcium, sodium, potassium, magnesium, & Vitamins A, B1, B2, and C; may aid digestion. |

✠ Condiments & Spices

Condiments are a great way to add great flavor to an otherwise basic dish. Many people are unaware of how many wonderful choices there are! Look for products that do not contain added sugars or other highly refined additives. Read labels, buy good quality, and, when possible, make them at home. Be creative and try new things! If you don't like it, that is ok—someone else in your family might!

Good to Know:

Experiment with and learn how to use herbs and spices. When herbs are dried, they are in concentrated form. One tablespoon of fresh herbs = one teaspoon of dry. Basil, cilantro, oregano, parsley, rosemary, and thyme are great for soups, stews, salads, and sauces and to season chicken, fish, and meats. Sweet spices, as mentioned earlier under healthy sweeteners, like cinnamon and nutmeg, are great for baking, desserts, warm breakfasts (like oatmeal), and in smoothies. Below is a great list of options for you to try.

CONDIMENTS

Condiment	The Good Stuff	
Basic Spices	Cinnamon* Curry powder* Ginger* Turmeric* Saffron* Thyme*	Cumin* Garlic* Oregano * Basil* Sage* Rosemary*
Peppers	Black Chili powder White pepper	Cayenne Chili Flakes
Salts	Sea salt	Herbamare
Oils	Chili oil Olive oil Flavored olive oils	Flaxseed oil Hot sesame oil Toasted sesame oil
Vinegars	Apple cider vinegar Red wine vinegar	Balsamic vinegar Umeboshi vinegar (plum)
Sauces	Bragg's amino acids Olive paste Salad dressings Tomato sauce	Hot sauces Pesto Tamari soy sauce
Sea vegetables (very nutritious)	Dulse flakes	Nori flakes
Other	Chutneys Ketchup (with no added sugar) Parmesan cheese Sauerkraut	Coconut milk Mustards Pickles Sprouts: alfalfa, sunflower, mung

* All of these spices have been shown to improve brain health and healing.

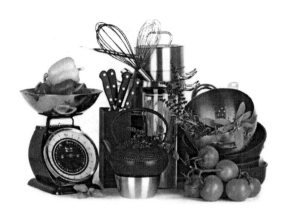

"I like a cook who smiles out loud when he tastes his own work. Let God worry about your modesty; I want to see your enthusiasm." – Robert Farrar Capon

CHAPTER 5

Recipes

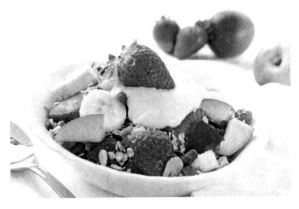

Breakfast

Breakfast is really important in the morning to get your body energized and your brain working to the best of its ability.

What We Love:

- ♥ Fruit & Vanilla Almond Milk Smoothies (shown in Beverage/Smoothie section)

- ♥ Gluten-Free Waffles with fruit and butter or a small amount of Trader Joe's Agave Nectar Maple Syrup Blend (We love Trader Joe's GF Waffles.)

- ♥ Nature's Path Gluten-Free Cereals: (www.naturespath.com) Organic Hemp Plus Granola, Organic Millet Rice, Organic Whole O's

- ♥ Hodgson Mill Gluten-Free Pancake and Waffle Mix (www.HodgsonMill.com) They also sell muffin mixes.

- ♥ Arrowhead Mills: (www.arrowheadmills.com) Organic Maple Buckwheat Flakes – They also sell GF All Purpose baking mix and other mixes.

- ♥ Envirokids (Part of Nature's Path) Organic Koala Crisp Cocoa Cereal (as a special treat)

- ♥ Natural Peanut Butter and sliced Banana on a Gluten-Free English muffin

- ♥ Think Thin Bars (www.thinkthinproducts.com) NO!! We do not eat these to lose weight; we eat them because they contain 15-20g of protein and NO sugar. My son eats one every day at school for a healthy snack. They taste great and come in many flavors—great for on the go!

Fruit Parfaits
1 serving

¼ c. GF granola
¼ c. plain or Greek yogurt
½ c. fruit of your choice
Cinnamon to taste

Place ½ of the granola in a small bowl or parfait dish. Add ½ of the yogurt mixed with cinnamon. Top with ½ of the fruit. Layer all again. It can be refrigerated for up to 2 hours.

Egg on a Muffin
1 serving

GF English Muffin – toasted
1 egg (local if possible)
1 piece of cheese of your preference

Sauté egg in ½ teaspoon coconut oil and flip. Top with cheese and any veggies that you like. Spread a little butter and any preferred condiments on the muffin and top with egg. Serve.

Green Eggs
1 serving

2 eggs
1 tbsp. water or milk
Dash of sea salt
1/2 c. baby spinach leaves
1/8 c. grated cheese of your choice

Whisk together eggs, milk, and salt in a bowl. Sauté eggs in ½ teaspoon coconut oil, flipping eggs when nearly cooked. Add the spinach and the cheese. Cover and remove from heat to wilt spinach (less than one minute). Serve. (Also would be good with salsa.)

Huevos Rancheros
4 servings

1 tbsp. extra-virgin olive oil
¼ onion, chopped
2-3 cloves garlic, minced
1 16oz. can diced tomatoes with green chilies
½ tsp. sea salt
½ tsp. chili powder
2 tsp. butter or coconut oil

Heat oil in a medium-size skillet. Add onion, garlic, tomatoes, salt, and chili powder. Bring to a boil. Reduce heat and simmer 5-7 minutes. Keep warm.

In a second frying pan, heat butter or coconut oil over low heat. Crack each egg into pan and cook covered for 3 minutes. Remove the cover and cook until yolk is almost set.

Each egg can be served atop a brown rice tortilla with warm sauce poured on top. Can be served with grated cheese or sour cream on top and avocado slices and black beans on the side.

Steel Cut Oats
1 serving

1 c. oatmeal or brown rice
¼ cup of walnuts
¼ c. of unsweetened vanilla almond milk or milk of your choice (If using soy, buy only Non-GMO)
½ tsp. brown sugar or natural sweetener
½ c. cubed apple or fruit of choice

Warm up milk, oatmeal, and walnuts. Add fruit before serving. You can also add cinnamon to taste. Experiment! You can add goji berries, sunflower seeds, grated ginger, etc.

*I purchase Trader Joe's Quick Cook (8 Minute) Steel Cut Oats and cook 5-6 servings ahead of time. **OR,** I substitute brown rice for the oatmeal instead. (Tastes great – really!) I cook a full pan of brown rice at the beginning of the week and use it for breakfast, lunch, or dinner.

Ezekiel Bread French Toast

2 servings

Because Ezekiel breads are from sprouted grains, they are allowed, even though they are not completely gluten free.

1 whole egg and one egg white, lightly beaten
Olive oil spray or 2 tsp. coconut oil
¼ tsp. vanilla
Pinch of sea salt
4 slices Ezekiel bread of choice
½ c. banana
6 oz. of plain yogurt
(can add cinnamon for flavor and sweetness)

Mix eggs, vanilla, and salt in a shallow, flat bowl. Preheat a large skillet to medium and add oil. Coat 2 pieces of bread in egg mixture on both sides until ½ of egg is absorbed. Place into skillet and cook until golden brown. Repeat with remaining bread slices. Put 2 slices of French toast on a plate and top with ½ of the yogurt and banana slices. Add additional fruit for sweetness if desired.

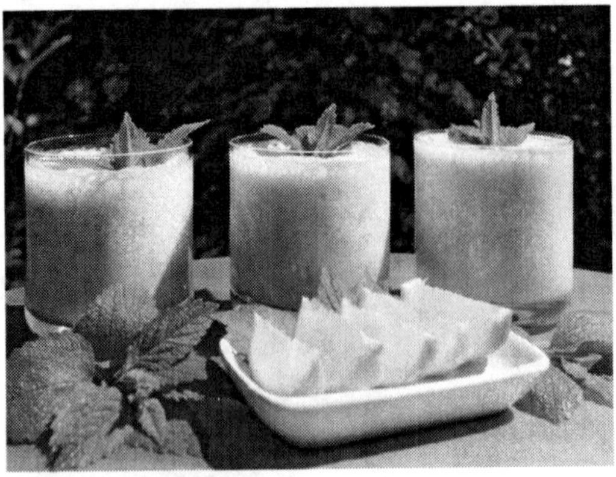

Beverages & Smoothies

Keeping yourself hydrated is KEY in recovering from Mild Traumatic Brain Injury and for the rest of us as well! Many individuals that are recovering from MTBI have problems with swallowing initially, so smoothies can be great in that transitional period without sacrificing nutrition.

Make sure that you have a powerful, good quality blender; it makes the job so much easier.

NOTE: To make many of the following smoothies complete nutritionally, add one scoop of high quality protein powder while blending.

What We Love:

- WATER, WATER, WATER—so important!! Be careful to read the labels of flavored waters because many contain additives or added sugars that are unnecessary and should be avoided.
- Hint Water (http://www.drinkhint.com/) is healthy water infused with natural flavors with no added sweeteners or calories. My son loves them, and I can feel good about it.

♥ Organic 2% milk--we don't drink milk on a regular basis ourselves, but we mix it into recipes and to thicken smoothies.

♥ Almond Breeze Unsweetened Vanilla Almond Milk (www. almondbreeze.com) is delightful! You would swear there was sugar in it! We use it as our primary milk for cereal, smoothies, and even in mashed potatoes! They also carry other flavors, both refrigerated and in aseptic shelf-stable packaging.

♥ If you need to drink coffee, drink ONLY Organic. Why? Because coffee is one of the most pesticide treated crops in the world. We love The Organic Coffee Company (http://www. organiccoffeecompany.com/). Their products are affordable and easily available at most local grocers.

♥ We don't drink many juices because of the sugar content. We do use a couple of Trader Joe's Carrot Juice Blends to mix liquid vitamins into.

♥ Polar Seltzers are good and unsweetened (http://www.polarbev. com/).

Banana Split Smoothie
1 serving

1 c. unsweetened almond milk (regular or vanilla)
1 ½ c. frozen banana slices
½ c. pineapple chunks
5 frozen strawberries
1 ½ tbsp. sweetened cocoa powder or Cacao powder (contains antioxidants)

Add milk to blender. Put cocoa powder in blender first followed by fruit. Blend until smooth.

Packs-a-Punch Raspberry Almond Smoothie
4 servings
(Courtesy of the Almond Board of California)

2 c. almond milk
1 12oz. package of frozen raspberries
2 medium bananas, cut into chunks
2 tsp. organic honey
½ tsp. almond extract

Combine all in a blender until smooth. May be garnished with whole almonds if desired.

Strawberry Lemonade Smoothie
1 serving
(Courtesy of Blue Diamond Growers)

6 oz. unsweetened vanilla almond milk
2 c. strawberries
1 tsp. lemon zest
3 tbsp. fresh lemon juice
1 tsp. natural sweetener (like Stevia)
3 ice cubes

Blend all together until smooth. Remember, for more nutritional value, add one scoop high-quality protein powder.

Mango Blues
1 serving

This drink is recommended for boosting your memory. It's also great for giving you energy and strengthening your immune system, and as a bonus, it is great for your skin!

2 mangoes (can be purchased frozen and already cubed)
2 handfuls of blueberries
Juice of one fresh lime
8 tbsp. apple juice

Blend well and serve immediately.

Creamy Green Banana
1 serving

This easy-to-make drink is recommended for people that are recovering from an injury. By the way, Spirulina is really good for you and easy to find in powdered form. (Make sure it's pure.)

What is Spirulina? It's blue-green algae that contains 18 vitamins and minerals, 100x's the Vitamin A of carrots, 50x's the iron of spinach, 7x's the calcium of milk, and 6x's the protein in eggs. (It doesn't taste bad!)

This drink gives you energy, boosts your immune system, and is great for digestion.

1 banana
¼ - ½ c. pineapple
1 tsp. spirulina
5 tbsp. regular or Greek yogurt
6 tbsp. pineapple juice

Blend well and serve immediately.

Joint Aid Smoothie
1 serving

All of the ingredients in this smoothie reduce inflammation in the body.

1 pineapple (can be purchased frozen or already chopped)
1 inch of ginger root
1 tbsp. flaxseed or coconut oil

Blend well and serve immediately. Add a little water if it is too thick.

My Favorite Smoothie
1 serving

I love this smoothie!I It's cleansing and contains healthy fats, and it is easy to make and tastes great. It's a great way to dip your taste buds into incorporating greens into your drinks! My clients love it, and they drink it often.

1 large handful of baby spinach leaves
1 ripe banana (frozen is great, but peel first and then freeze.)
½ of a lemon, deseeded (can use only the juice if you prefer)
½ of an avocado
½ - 1 tsp. of flax seed
1 c. pineapple
1/3 of a seeded cucumber
¾ c. of filtered water

Blend and serve immediately.

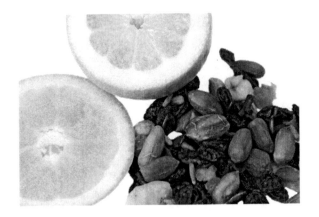

✖ Snacks

There is nothing wrong with snacking, as long as it is done in moderation, and you train yourself to make healthy, tasty choices!

What We Love:

♥ Simply Fruit Roll-Ups

   Unlike regular fruit-roll ups that are made by the same company, these are 90% real fruit and fruit juice, and they don't taste like cardboard. Plus, you can purchase them at your local market easily. Only one a day is allowed because they contain sugar.

♥ Glutino Gluten-Free Pretzels

   This company has many gluten-free snacks to pick from (http://www.glutino.com/).

♥ Pirate Brands gluten-free snacks

   We like "Tings," the crunchy corn sticks are the best (http://piratebrands.com/).

♥ Mary's Gone Crackers Black Pepper Crackers

My son loves these spread with a little cream cheese

(http://www.marysgonecrackers.com/ns/intro.php).

♥ Crunchmaster Crackers

These are similar to Mary's Gone Crackers above, but with other flavor options (http://www.crunchmaster.com/home. aspx).

♥ Organic Corn Tortilla Chips

Serve with hummus or salsa for a tasty treat.

♥ Any kind of fruit or veggies, peeled and chopped up—

Do it ahead of time and always have some on hand so that you don't reach for the less than optimal stuff.

♥ Smoothies mentioned in the Smoothie section and the Think Thin bars under the Breakfast Section

♥ Square of dark chocolate (YUM!)

♥ Other snack ideas to follow after featured recipes

Veggie Muffins
6 muffins

1 c. veggies, grated and finely chopped (your choice)
2 eggs, beaten
1 tbsp. natural sweetener (like Stevia)
2 cups gluten-free flour
¼- ½ c. finely chopped parsley
1 c. milk of your choice (Unsweetened vanilla almond milk would
be great here.)
Pinch of sea salt

Preheat oven to 325 degrees. Mix flour, salt, and sweetener in a bowl, making a well in the middle. Add eggs, veggies, and parsley. Mix, while gradually adding milk. It is supposed to be lumpy. Spoon into a muffin pan that has been oiled. Bake for 12-15 minutes. Remove and allow to set for 10 minutes before serving.

These are a great way to get those veggies in painlessly, and the parsley is good for digestion, too!

Mushroom and Onion Dip
12 servings

1 12oz. package of light cream cheese, softened
1 tsp. dried parsley
2 tsp. olive or coconut oil
2 c. sliced mushrooms, washed
½ c. diced red onions
2 tsp. ground black pepper

Because the mushrooms and onions are hot, it melts the cream cheese while mixing. You can serve this with gluten-free crackers or raw veggie sticks.

In a medium bowl, mix parsley and cream cheese. In a medium skillet over medium heat, warm oil. Add mushrooms, onions, and pepper. Cook 5-7 minutes until soft, stirring often. Pour hot mushrooms over cream cheese mixture and mix gently. Serve. (Remember, this serves 12!)

Apple Sandwiches with Granola and Peanut Butter
2 servings

2 small apples, cored and cut crosswise into ½ inch rounds
1 tsp. lemon juice
3 tbsp. almond, peanut, or cashew butter
2 tbsp. dark chocolate chips
3 tbsp. gluten-free granola

If you're not going to eat these immediately, brush apples with lemon juice to prevent them from turning brown. Spread peanut butter on 1 piece of the apple, sprinkling with granola and chocolate chips. Put another apple piece on top, pushing down gently to distribute spread. Serve.

These are really easy to make. If you don't have an apple corer, slice the apples into rounds, and cut out the center. If you wrap these tightly, you can eat them on the go!

Quick and Spicy Tamari Nut Mix
Makes 3 ½ cups

2 tsp. peanut or coconut oil
1 c. shelled pumpkin seeds
1 c. shelled peanuts
½ c. cashews
½ c. walnuts or pecans
½ c. almonds
1 tbsp. soy sauce or tamari
1/8 tsp. cayenne pepper
Squeeze of fresh lemon

This can be served warm or at room temperature. Cayenne is a great anti-inflammatory spice. You can adjust the spiciness to your taste.

Heat oil in a large sauté pan on medium heat. Add nuts, stirring often, until they appear golden brown. Drizzle soy sauce over the mixture. Add cayenne and a squeeze of lemon, stirring thoroughly. Cool for 15 minutes and then serve. This can be stored for up to one week.

Gluten-Free Chex Style Mix
8 servings

According to people that eat it, it tastes as good as the original.

9 c. gluten-free Cinnamon Chex style rice cereal
2 c. gluten-free pretzels
1 c. pecans or nuts of your choice
8 tbsp. olive oil or coconut oil (liquefied)
1 tbsp. Worcestershire sauce
1-2 tsp. sea salt

Heat oven to 250 degrees. Mix oil, Worcestershire sauce, and seasonings in a bowl and blend. Place nuts, cereal, and pretzels in a large roasting pan. Add seasoning mix and coat mixture thoroughly. Bake uncovered in a preheated oven for 1 hour, stirring every 15 minutes. Cool and serve.

Tasty Fruit Salsa
8 servings

This dish is spicy and sweet together, and it's really easy to make quickly. This can be served with good quality corn chips or as a side dish with dinner.

1 10oz. can of chopped tomatoes and chilies
1 apple, unpeeled and diced
¼ c. bell pepper of your choice, chopped
¼ c. dried apricots, chopped

In a medium-sized bowl, mix all together and chill for 2 hours before serving. If you like, you can substitute other dried or fresh fruit of your choice for the apricots; like mango, strawberries, pears, etc

Other Healthy & Tasty Snack Ideas:

♥   Greek or plain yogurt with fruit

♥   Ezekiel bread with all fruit jam

♥   Olives

♥   Salted edamame (Soybean pods, cooked)

♥   Cheese

♥   Leftover soups

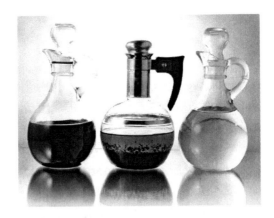

▓ Dressings & Sauces

You can really change up the flavor of your food by adding great dressings and sauces to your repertoire. Don't be afraid to experiment with new flavors; if it doesn't work out, that's ok. If you choose to not make your dressings/sauces, please be sure to read the ingredient label well.

Do not buy anything with partially hydrogenated oils, trans-fats, or food colorings. Don't forget to go back to the condiment section in the last chapter for some great ideas! Here are some wonderful options for you to try.

What We Love:

♥ Newman's Own Balsamic Vinaigrette

This easy-to-find dressing can be used as a marinade for chicken and veggies for the grill, on a multitude of salads, and drizzled over just cooked vegetables instead of heavy sauces. All of our guests always comment on how good it tastes. Additionally, all of the profits go to charity!

♥ Trader Joe's Spicy Peanut Vinaigrette

(It's not completely Gluten-Free, so use it in moderation.) It's not really spicy, and it is amazing on grains and veggies. Trader Joe's also has many other good dressings to suit your taste.

♥ Trader Joe's Hummus (many varieties available) and Tahini Both are great for a dip or as a sandwich spread.

Apple Salsa
4 servings

3 apples, peeled, cored, and seeded
1 medium sweet onion, diced
¼ c. fresh cilantro, chopped
1 tbsp. mint, chopped (less if you use dried)
2 tsp. lime juice
¼. c. flaxseed or olive oil
1 tbsp. agave nectar (or maple syrup as a special treat)

Mix all ingredients together and serve.

If the apples by themselves are too bland, mix in 1/2 c. of your favorite regular salsa. This tastes better if you make it a day before you serve it. If you like a smooth salsa, put half of the mixture into a blender for a couple of seconds. This is good with baked chips or grilled veggies.

Peanut Sauce
Makes 2 cups

1 c. natural peanut butter
¼ c. orange juice
1 tbsp. toasted sesame oil
1 tbsp. tamari (dark soy sauce – sometimes contains gluten)
dash cayenne pepper

Combine all ingredients in a bowl and mix with a fork. Add water in 1 tbsp. increments to reach desired consistency.

Avocado "Butter"
2-3 servings

2 tsp. fresh lime juice
1 very ripe avocado
Sea salt to taste

Pour lime juice in a small bowl. Scoop out avocado into lime juice and add salt.

Mash with a fork well and serve immediately. You can use this as a sandwich spread or as a dip for GF crackers or veggies. Great healthy fats!

Amazing Gravy
4 servings

2 c. broth
2 tbsp. GF flour
Salt and pepper to taste

This tasty gravy takes 10 minutes, and it uses only 2 ingredients. The quality of the flavor is determined by using a good quality broth by a company such as Imagine or Trader Joe's. Pick the flavor of your choice. They are usually sold in 1 quart boxes that have a very long shelf life so that you can keep them on hand.

In a medium saucepan, heat broth until it is very hot, but not boiling. Place flour in a small bowl and add enough broth to dissolve flour (about ¼ cup). Beat this with a wire whisk and then pour it back into the hot broth. Continue to whisk all broth while cooking over medium heat for 5-8 minutes, until lightly thickened. Add salt and pepper to taste. It can be stored in a tightly covered jar in the refrigerator.

French Lentil Dijon Spread
Makes 1 cup

2 tbsp. walnuts
1 c. cooked lentils
2 mushrooms, sliced
1 clove garlic
1 scallion, sliced
1 tbsp. whole grain mustard
1 tbsp. tamari (dark soy sauce)
½ tsp. pepper
Water

French lentils are tiny, black lentils that have a great taste. You can purchase them already cooked and vacuum packed at Trader Joe's and probably other retailers as well. You can eat this on a sandwich with lettuce, tomato, and mayo or as a party dip for crackers and veggies as well.

Grind walnuts in a blender or coffee grinder, or chop finely on a cutting board. Place all ingredients into a blender or food processor and mix until smooth. Add water to get the consistency you want. This will keep in the refrigerator for several days.

Yogurt Garlic Dip
Makes 1 cup

1 small or ½ large cucumber, peeled, seeded, and grated or
chopped fine in a processor
1 tsp. sea salt
1 c. whole milk yogurt, plain
1 clove garlic, minced
2 tsp. lemon juice
2 tbsp. chopped parsley

Place cucumber and salt in a dish. Place remaining ingredients in a bowl. Let each mixture set 5-10 minutes. Blend together and serve. This can be refrigerated for a couple of days.

This dip can be served with salmon, chicken, beef, or tofu. It can also be used with vegetables as well.

<u>The Best Pesto</u>
Makes 1 cup

3 garlic cloves, peeled
3 c. fresh basil leaves, packed down in cup
¾ - 1 c. fresh parsley leaves, packed down in cup
¼ c. pine nuts
1/3 – ½ c. extra virgin olive oil
1/3 c. grated parmesan or romano cheese
Sea salt and pepper to taste

Using parsley in this recipe helps to preserve the green color, and it's also a very cleansing herb. Extra virgin olive oil provides healthy Omega 3's for healing. This can be served over pasta, as a topping for chicken or fish, or even in soup.

Place garlic cloves in the bottom of food processor and chop. Add the basil and parsley leaves and chop. While the motor is running, add the nuts and the olive oil. Add the cheese and process again. If it is dry, add a little more olive oil. Season with salt and pepper to taste.

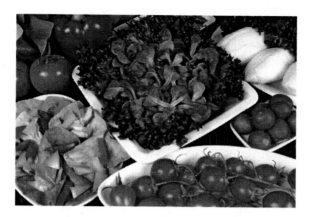

✠ Salads & Veggie Dishes

As you already know by now, greens and vegetables provide you with energy and many of the essential vitamins and minerals your body needs to function well. Here are several options for you to experiment with and enjoy.

What We Love:

♥ Bok Choy, washed, with ends cut and sliced into 1-2 inch pieces. We sauté it with one clove of minced garlic, ½ of a chopped onion, and 2 tsp. olive oil or coconut oil. Because of its high water content, it cooks quickly—under 10 minutes. Cook covered, stirring often. Add salt and pepper to taste. It's a great, quick side dish. (Bok Choy has long celery-like white stalks and dark green leaves at the top. It's loaded with calcium, Vitamins A, C, and E, and folic acid.)

♥ Big chunks of veggies put on skewers brushed in olive oil on the upper part of the grill. Yum!

Mashed Sweet Potatoes
3-4 servings

3 medium sweet potatoes, peeled and cut into 2-inch chunks
3 carrots, peeled, and cut into 1-2 inch pieces (for added sweetness)
½ - ¾ c. unsweetened vanilla almond milk or milk of your choice
2-3 tsp. of butter
1-2 tbsp. natural sweetener
Sea salt and pepper to taste

Boil sweet potatoes and carrots in a large pot of water for 15-20 minutes until tender. Drain. Add remaining ingredients and mash until smooth.

Minty Fresh Cucumber Salad
4 servings

2 cucumbers, washed, peeled, and thinly sliced
1 green apple, very thinly sliced
1 handful fresh mint
1-3 pinches of sea salt
Juice of ½ of a lemon

Rub salt into cucumber and apple slices. Finely chop mint and mix with cucumber and apple. Cover and let set in the refrigerator for 30 minutes. Add lemon juice and serve.

Portobello Mushroom Steaks
4 servings

4 portobello mushrooms
3 tsp. oregano
2 tbsp. balsamic vinegar
2 tbsp. olive oil
Sea salt and pepper to taste

Preheat oven to 350. Cut off mushroom stems and wash tops; pat dry with a towel. Mix oil, vinegar and oregano in a dish. Put mushrooms in a baking dish with an edge. Pour oil mixture over mushrooms and bake for 30 minutes. As an alternative, you can cook these on the grill by flipping them often and basting them with the oil mixture.

Sautéed Broccoli
4 servings

1 bunch broccoli, washed and cut into bite-sized pieces
½ c. grated carrot
¼ c. toasted sesame seeds
(Can substitute sesame seeds with another
healthy seed of your choice.)
1-2 tbsp. olive oil or coconut oil
Sea salt and black pepper

Warm oil in the pan, add broccoli stalk pieces, and sauté for a couple of minutes. Add broccoli florets and sauté for another 2 minutes. Add 3 tbsp. water and add grated carrots. Cover and steam for 3-4 minutes. Remove from heat. Add sesame seeds, salt, and pepper. Serve.

Arugula Walnut Salad
4-6 servings

4-5 tbsp. lightly toasted walnut pieces
2 bunches arugula leaves (about 4 cups), washed and torn into
bite sized pieces
1 -1 ½ c. shredded radicchio
1 yellow pepper, sliced into thin strips
3 tbsp. olive oil
2 tbsp. minced red onion
1/8 - 1/4 tsp. sea salt
1 tbsp. minced fresh parsley, or 1 tsp. dried
1 tbsp. balsamic vinegar
¼ c. orange juice

Heat oven to 325. Place walnuts on a cookie sheet and toast for 3-5 minutes. Check walnuts often to make sure they do not burn. Place arugula into medium sized bowl. Add radicchio, pepper, and cooled walnuts to arugula and toss. Set aside. In small skillet, heat 1 tbsp. of the olive oil. Add red onion and cook for 5 minutes. Sprinkle salt over onion and add parsley. Stir. Just before serving, add remaining oil and vinegar and heat through. Remove from heat and add orange juice. Pour over salad, toss gently, and serve immediately.

The nutty taste of the arugula and walnuts are enhanced by the warm, orange balsamic vinaigrette.

It also looks great!

Stir-Fry Napa Cabbage
Serves 3-4

1 small head napa cabbage, or 6-7 cups chopped (You can also purchase already shredded.)

1 carrot, peeled and cut into matchstick pieces (You can buy this shredded also.)

3 scallions, thinly sliced (Use mostly the green parts only.)

1 tsp. olive oil or coconut oil

1 tbsp. minced ginger or 1 tsp. dried

Pinch of sea salt

1 handful of cilantro leaves

½ - 1 tsp. dark sesame oil

2 tbsp. sesame seeds, toasted

If not purchased shredded, cut cabbage into quarters and slice thinly. Cut carrot into round pieces and slice into matchsticks— or use the equivalent amount in shredded carrot (about ¼ cup). Heat a wok or skillet over medium-high heat. Add oil and coat the pan. Add ginger and carrot and stir-fry for 1 minute. Add cabbage and salt, cooking for 2-3 minutes to remain crisp, or cook a little longer if you like it softer. Remove pan from stove and add scallions and cilantro leaves. Add sesame oil and sesame seeds, and mix thoroughly. Serve immediately.

Mediterranean Crunch Salad
4 servings

(Courtesy of the Whole Foods website)

1 15oz. can of garbanzo beans, rinsed thoroughly
1 cucumber, peeled and chopped
1 c. broccoli, florets, chopped
1 c. grape tomatoes, halved
1 c. finely sliced kale – or green of your choice
½ c. finely chopped red onion
2 tbsp. finely chopped black olives
3 tbsp. each red wine vinegar and olive oil
1 small clove garlic, minced
1 tbsp. fresh parsley (or ½-1 tsp. dried)
1 tbsp. fresh thyme (or ½-1 tsp. dried)

Combine all ingredients in a large bowl and chill 1 hour before serving.

This salad is great on its own, on top of a gluten-free bagel for lunch, or with chicken or shrimp on top as a meal.

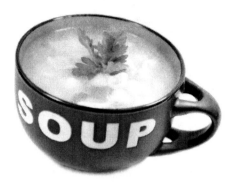

❇ Soups

Soups are a great way to take in multiple nutrients quickly. Here are some easy-to-make ideas for you to try. Once it's done, you have many servings or enough for a small crowd.

What We Love:

♥ Trader Joe's Vegetable, Free-Range Chicken and Beef Broths— They do NOT contain any MSG or un-natural ingredients. Because they are in aseptic packaging, they have a long shelf life.

♥ Vogue Cuisine Instant Flavored Bases

They have chicken, onion, beef, and vegetarian. They are gluten-free and low sodium and all natural, and they contain non-GMO soy ingredients. It can be used in place of stock/broth by mixing with water. Check out their website for many other uses: http://www.voguecuisine.com/gluten-free-low-sodium-base.html.

Three Sisters Stew
6-8 servings

Native Americans grew corn, beans, and squash together, and thus, they are called "the three sisters." This dish is great for chilly evenings. If you use delicata squash, there is no need to peel it.

2 cans lima beans, rinsed thoroughly
2-3 c. vegetable or chicken broth
1-1 ½ tsp. ground cumin
1 tbsp. olive oil or coconut oil
2 tsp. oregano, dried
½ tsp. cinnamon
1 medium onion, chopped
2 tsp. sea salt
3 cloves garlic, minced
2-3 c. squash, peeled and cut into chunks
1 14oz. can chopped tomatoes
1 tsp. chili powder
1 c. corn
½ c. grated cheese for garnish

Heat a pasta sized pot to medium, add oil, cumin, oregano, and cinnamon and sauté for 30 seconds. Add onion, salt, and garlic and cook until onion is soft. Add squash, tomatoes, and chili powder, bring to a simmer and cook until squash is soft (about 20 minutes). Add broth, beans, and corn. Adjust seasoning for your taste. Serve hot with grated cheese on top.

<u>Lentil Soup</u>
4-6 servings

This is an easy way to get your veggies in, and it tastes great with the red wine vinegar.

¼ c. finely chopped onion
¼ c. chopped celery
½ c. diced pepper (red, green, yellow or orange)
½ tsp. olive oil
1 garlic clove, minced
¼ tsp. dried parsley
¼ tsp. sea salt
1 c. dried lentils
3 cups filtered water
½ c. shredded zucchini
½ c. shredded carrots
¼ c. chopped spinach
1 tbsp. red wine vinegar (you can use cider vinegar for a slightly different flavor)

In a large pot over medium heat, sauté onion, celery, and pepper in olive oil until soft. Add garlic, parsley, salt, lentils, and water. Bring to a boil, reduce heat, and simmer 20 minutes. Add zucchini and carrots and simmer for 10 minutes. Add spinach and red wine vinegar and simmer for 3 minutes. Serve.

Chicken Noodle Soup with Vegetables
6-8 servings

1 lb. chicken breast, cut into 1 inch pieces
¼ c, diced onions
2 tbsp. olive or coconut oil
¼ c. shredded carrots
¼ c. diced pepper of choice
1/8 tsp. garlic powder
1 bay leaf
1/8 tsp. dried thyme
1/8 tsp. sea salt
1/8 tsp. black pepper
3 c. water or chicken broth (or filtered water)
2 c. brown rice pasta
1 c. broccoli florets

This is a delicious blend of chicken, vegetables, and herbs. You can use brown rice pasta, brown rice, or even quinoa. If you prefer, cook the noodles/rice ahead of time according to their directions. Place a portion into each bowl and then add this soup on top. This prevents the pasta/rice from getting mushy.

In a large pot over medium-high heat, sauté chicken and onions in olive oil for 10 minutes. Add carrots, pepper, garlic powder, bay leaf, thyme, salt, and pepper. Stir 2 minutes and add broth. Bring to a boil. Reduce heat to medium. Add noodles and broccoli and simmer 8-10 minutes. Remove bay leaf and serve.

Italian White Bean Soup with Broccoli Rabe
2 ½ quarts

The garlic adds yummy flavor to the beans and potatoes. Garlic is a great addition to any dish and is naturally anti-inflammatory and anti-bacterial—great for healing and tasty too! This dish takes 45-60 minutes to prepare.

1 c. dried white navy or great northern beans (soaked overnight)
4 medium red potatoes, peeled and diced
1 bay leaf
2 whole celery stalks
8 c. cold water
2 tbsp. olive oil
1 large onion, chopped
1 leek, washed, sliced (using white parts only)
3 carrots, peeled and diced
1 pound broccoli rabe, (about 6 cups, chopped)
4 garlic cloves, minced
1 hot red pepper, minced or 1/8 tsp. red pepper flakes

Drain beans and discard water. Place beans, potatoes, bay leaf, and whole celery stalks in a large soup pot with 8 cups of water and bring to a boil. Lower the heat, cover, and simmer for 30 minutes. (The celery stalks add flavor and will be discarded like the bay leaf when the soup is done.)

In a large skillet, heat 1 tbsp. oil and sauté onion and leeks for 8-10 minutes. Add carrots and sauté for 2-3 minutes. Add mixture to beans and simmer for another 20-30 minutes.

While the soup cooks, wash chopped broccoli rabe well. Heat remaining tbsp. of oil in skillet and add minced garlic and red pepper. Cook 1 minute. Add chopped rabe and 2-3 tbsp. of water. Cover and cook for 5-8 minutes. When the beans are tender, add the cooked rabe, and cook for 5 minutes to allow all flavors to mix together. Remove bay leaf and celery stalks.

Easy Hamburger Soup
8-10 servings

My mom gave me this recipe, and I added a couple of things. It's a one-pot recipe—can't get any easier than that!

1- 1 ½ lb. good quality ground beef
1 medium onion, chopped
1 16oz. can chopped tomatoes
2 c. water
1 aseptic box of chicken or beef broth (with no MSG)
1 can of healthy tomato soup
4 carrots, chopped
3-4 stalks celery, chopped
1 clove garlic, minced
2 c. baby spinach leaves
1 bay leaf
2 tbsp. fresh parsley or 1 ½ tsp. dried
½ tsp. thyme
½ c. quinoa or brown rice
Sea salt and pepper to taste

Brown meat and drain well; set aside. Place browned meat in large pot and add all other ingredients, except spinach leaves. Simmer for 1 ½ hrs. Ten minutes before serving, add spinach, stirring often.

Serve as is or add a little shredded cheese as a topping on each bowl. This soup can be frozen as well.

Santa Fe Stew
10-12 servings

Want to spice it up a little, but not too much? Then this is right up your alley. It's chock full of flavor and the cumin and chili powder are great anti-inflammatory spices. Enjoy!

1 ½ lb. good quality ground turkey
3 lg. onions, chopped
6-8 large carrots, chopped
1 can black beans, rinsed well
1 can kidney beans, rinsed well
1 can cannellini beans, rinsed well
1 can tomatoes with green chilies, undrained
2-3 cans diced tomatoes, undrained
1 can corn, rinsed well
4 c. chicken broth, (with no MSG)
1 tsp. chili powder
1-2 tsp. ground cumin
1 tsp. black pepper
½. tsp. ground red pepper or red pepper flakes
2 tbsp. dried herbs of choice (like oregano, basil, etc.)
1/2 tsp. coconut oil or cooking spray

Coat a large pot with coconut oil or cooking spray. Cook turkey until lightly browned, about 8 minutes, stirring often. Add onions and carrots. Cook for another 5 minutes. Add all of the remaining ingredients, stirring well. Simmer for 2 hours, uncovered. If end result is too thick, add a little water. Serve alone or over cooked brown rice or grain of your choice.

Green Power Soup
4-6 servings

This is a great way to get your greens in, and it is an easy, healthy choice. I'm not kidding—it really tastes good! My clients really like it. (It gives you serious energy.) You need a good blender or food processor for this one.

1 small onion, chopped
1 large zucchini, washed and cut into ½ pieces
2 c. broccoli florets
2 c. asparagus, chopped (throw ends away)
1 c. kale, collard greens, spinach or greens of your choice
1 tsp. dry granulated garlic
5 c. chicken broth or water
Sea salt and pepper to taste
Butter or coconut oil for serving

Put all ingredients into a large pot. Bring to a boil, reduce heat, cover, and simmer until vegetables are fork tender and bright in color, but not overcooked (about 5-6 minutes). Puree soup in small batches in a blender and pour into large bowl to hold. Return all of pureed soup to pot, adding 2-3 pats of butter or 2-3 tbsp. of coconut oil to add flavor (1 tbsp. for each 2 cups of soup.) The fat from the butter actually allows your body to absorb the nutrients in the veggies better. Taste and adjust seasonings. Serve soup warm.

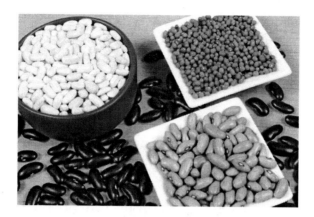

🞊 Beans & Grains

Both beans and grains in their natural state contain complex carbohydrates, protein, fiber, unsaturated fats, and a multitude of vitamins and minerals. They both can be prepared in bulk in advance and stored in the refrigerator for use throughout the week. Remember to go back to the "grains" section to experiment with different kinds.

What We Love:

♥ Brown Rice

I make a large batch of brown rice usually on a Sunday afternoon as I am preparing lunch for my family. It takes about 30 minutes to cook, and then it is available all week for breakfast (yes!), lunch, and dinner. I have it for breakfast mixed with walnuts, apples, and unsweetened vanilla almond milk, for lunch mixed with salad or leftovers, and for a variety of options for dinner.

♥ Trader Joe's vacuum packed Black Beluga Lentils

These can be found in the refrigerated section. They are full of protein, taste great, and are ready to go.

♥ Quinoa (Keen-wah)

This great tasting grain is easy to cook and contains more protein than any other grain. It also can be eaten either hot or cold. It is very versatile, because it takes on the flavor of whatever you prepare it with.

Quinoa Salad with Green Onion Vinaigrette
6 servings

In this recipe, you can stick with the quinoa or use the grain of your choice that is already prepared (like brown rice pasta, wild brown rice, etc.)

1 c. quinoa
½ small red onion, diced
2 plum tomatoes, diced
1 c. finely chopped fresh parsley
½ c. finely chopped fresh mint leaves
4 green onions, sliced, plus
½ c. chopped green onions
¼ c. lime juice
1 tbsp. honey
1 serrano chile pepper, chopped
½ c. olive oil
1 tsp. sea salt
½ tsp. black pepper

Place quinoa in a large bowl, pour 2 cups boiling water on top, cover the bowl tightly, and let it sit for 15-20 minutes. Drain well, squeezing out as much water as possible. In the bowl, mix quinoa with onion, tomatoes, parsley, mint, and 4 sliced green onions. Place the lime juice, honey, serrano pepper, and ½ c. chopped green onion in a blender and blend until smooth. With the motor running, add oil until fully mixed. If it is too thick, add a few tablespoons of water. Add salt and pepper to taste. Drizzle the quinoa salad with the green onion vinaigrette and serve.

Brown Basmati Pilaf
4 servings

Basmati adds a sweet flavor to the already nutritious brown rice, and it makes a quick and easy side dish.

1 c. brown basmati rice
½ c. dried cranberries
½ c. walnut pieces
½ c. chopped fresh parsley
2 cups water
Sea salt to taste
Add olive oil (if desired)

Rinse rice in a fine mesh strainer. Boil the water and add rice and salt. After 15 minutes, add cranberries and walnuts on top. Do not stir. Cook 15-20 more minutes, until all liquid is absorbed. Remove from heat, add parsley, and mix all ingredients. If desired, drizzle olive oil in. Serve.

<u>Orange and Walnut Quinoa</u>
4 servings

These flavors are great together. You get great Omega 3's from the walnuts, too.

1 ½ c. quinoa
Zest of 2 navel oranges (You can serve the oranges after dinner.)
½ c. chopped walnuts
2 ½ c. chicken or vegetable broth
2 tbsp. flat leaf parsley, chopped or 1 tsp. dried
1-2 tbsp. olive oil

Rinse quinoa in fine mesh strainer. Combine broth, oil, and quinoa in a pot and bring to a boil. Cover, lowering heat to simmer, and cook for 12 minutes. Remove from heat and let stand for 5 minutes. Stir quinoa and add orange zest, parsley, and walnuts. Serve.

Black Bean Extravaganza
4 servings

This dish can be served as a side dish, with grains or with greens. If you want to save an hour of cooking time, use canned beans, rinsing thoroughly. This is a great anti-inflammatory dish.

4 c. black beans
1 bell pepper of your choice, deseeded and chopped small
1 onion diced
1 lime
¾ c. water or broth
½ c. cilantro, chopped
2-3 cloves garlic, minced
2 tbsp. cinnamon
2 tsp. cumin
1 tbsp. olive oil
1 tsp. sea salt
Pinch of cayenne pepper

If starting with dried beans, soak 2 cups overnight. Rinse, place in a pot with 3 ½ c. of water, and bring to a boil. Add cinnamon and cumin and cook for 1 hour. If using canned beans, rinse them well, add them to a large pot, mix with spices, and add water or broth. Cover and cook over medium heat for 10 minutes. In a skillet, sauté onions, garlic, and oil. Mix beans with onion mixture, raw peppers, cayenne, and salt. (If you do not like raw peppers, you can sauté them with the onion). Garnish with cilantro and a wedge of lime to squeeze on top. Serve.

Mediterranean Quinoa
4 servings

This protein and amino-acid rich dish is wonderful, and the herbs help with digestion. This would go great with chicken or fish or on its own for a quick lunch on the go.

1 c. quinoa
1 ¾ c. water
½ tsp. sea salt
¼ c. toasted pine nuts
¼ c. lemon juice
¼ c. olive oil
3 tbsp. fresh mint, or 1 ½ tsp. dried
3 tbsp. chopped fresh parsley or 1 ½ tsp. dried
3 scallions
¼ c. currants
1/3 c. crumbled feta cheese

Rinse and drain quinoa in a mesh strainer. Place in a large pot with water and salt. Bring to a boil, then lower heat and simmer 15-20 minutes until all liquid is absorbed. Do not stir while it is cooking. Remove lid and set aside for 5-10 minutes. While quinoa is cooking, dry-toast pine nuts in skillet on low heat until they start to get light brown and give off an aroma (about 10 minutes). Combine olive oil, lemon juice, mint, and parsley in a large bowl. Add scallions, currants, feta cheese, and pine nuts and toss. Add warm quinoa slowly, tossing often. Serve at room temperature.

Golden Spice Rice with Chickpeas
4 servings

Adding grains and beans together gives you double nutritional value. When you sauté the rice before you cook it, it makes it less sticky.

2 tbsp. butter, olive oil, or coconut oil
1 c. brown basmati rice, rinsed and drained
¼ tsp. turmeric
1 ¾ - 2 c. water
½ tsp. cardamom
½ tsp. sea salt
1 cup cooked chickpeas
½ c. frozen green peas
¼ c. currants

Heat 2 tsp. butter in a medium-sized pan over medium heat. Add rice and sauté until well coated with butter. Add turmeric and stir. Add water, cardamom, and salt. Bring to a boil. Turn heat to low, so it is lightly simmering. Cover pan and let cook for 45-50 minutes or until all water is absorbed. Heat the remaining butter in large skillet over medium heat. Add chickpeas, peas, and currants and stir. Add rice, stirring often. Serve warm.

Nutty Brown Rice Burgers
8 small burgers

The apples and pecans sweeten the burgers and the salsa gives it a kick. Happy tastebuds!

1 cup cooked brown rice
1 cup diced apple
1 can black beans, drained and rinsed
½ c. chopped pecans (or nut of your choice – we like chopped walnuts)
¼ c. shredded carrots
1/3 c. salsa
1 tbsp. olive or coconut oil
Swiss or cheddar cheese (optional)
1 egg
½ c. gluten-free bread crumbs

In a large bowl, combine rice, apple, pecans, carrots, salsa, egg, and breadcrumbs. Mix well. Place beans in another bowl, mashing them completely. (You can add a tsp. of olive oil to assist this process.) Combine beans with other ingredients until all ingredients stick together. In a large skillet over medium heat, warm oil. Spoon about ¾ c. of rice mixture into skillet, flattening with the back of spoon to shape into a patty. (You can use an ice cream scoop to put mixture into pan.) Cook 5 minutes, turning once. Keep patties warm in the oven until they are complete. You can serve solo with a green salad or on gluten-free rolls or English muffins topped with cheese. We prefer them without the rolls because they still tend to fall apart.

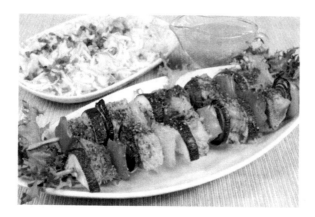

✠ Main Dishes

There is a whole WORLD of options for you in this area. Remember to use all of the resources available to you in the "Wonderful Foods That You Can Eat" chapter, and use your imagination!

What We Love - (when you don't have much time):

- ♥ Trader Joe's Black Bean & Corn Enchiladas

  They are dairy and wheat-free and are not too spicy.

- ♥ Bell & Evans Gluten-Free Breaded Chicken

  There are many options for a quick meal (www.bellandevans. com).

- ♥ Barber Foods "Seasoned Selects" No-Batter Stuffed Chicken Breasts

  We like the Broccoli & Cheese option. These contain less than 2% of wheat (www.barberfoods.com).

- ♥ Brown Rice Pasta

  Cook with 1 tsp. of oil in water to prevent sticking. Mix with

Tomato Basil Pasta Sauce. Sprinkle with shredded cheese and serve with a quick salad.

♥ Grilled cheese on a good gluten-free or Ezekiel bread

Healthy Slow-Cooker Stew
4-6 servings

Prepare it in the morning, and it's ready to enjoy at dinner time! You can add sliced greens as a variation 30 minutes before serving.

1 pound cubed beef
1 c. cubed turnip
2 medium red potatoes, cubed
1 medium onion, chopped
2 garlic cloves, minced
3 large carrots, sliced
2 bay leaves
2 tsp. dried thyme
3 tbsp. tomato paste
½ tsp. celery salt
½ tsp black pepper
1 quart beef broth (without MSG)

Place the meat, seasonings, vegetables, and broth in a slow cooker/crock-pot. Cover and cook on low for 6-8 hours. Remove the bay leaves and serve.

Brown Rice Tortilla Pizza
1 serving
(My son eats 2 at a time.)

This is an easy, tasty way to make a quick meal. Add a couple of ingredients, and you are good to go. Use the ingredients that are featured here, or pick your favorites—just about anything will work.

2 brown rice tortillas
1 tsp. coconut oil or olive oil
4 tbsp. pasta sauce
½ c. (or so) baby spinach leaves
¼ c. chopped sweet onion
1/3 of a plum tomato, seeded, and chopped
¼ c. shredded cheese

Preheat oven to 350. While oven is preheating, sauté onion in oil. Place tortillas on cookie sheet. Do NOT put any oil on the brown rice tortilla as it makes it mushy. Add 2 tsp. of sauce to each tortilla, spreading it around to the edges with the back of a soup spoon. Stir onions as they finish cooking. Place baby spinach leaves and chopped tomato pieces on each pizza. Add onions and shredded cheese. Bake for 10 minutes. Wait 1 minute, slice, and serve.

Tuna Steaks with Cucumber Dill Salsa
4 servings

4 tuna steaks (try to purchase US Albacore tuna)
½ of a large cucumber
1 c. purple kale (or other green of choice)
2 tbsp. fresh dill or 1 tbsp. dried
3 tbsp. olive oil
1 tbsp. red wine vinegar
Sea salt and pepper

Scoop out seeds from the cucumber. Dice and mix with the dill and the kale. Heat a skillet over medium-high heat. Rub a bit of olive oil on tuna steaks and cook for 3-4 minutes on each side. Time will vary due to thickness and your preference.

Place tuna steaks on plates and top with salsa. Keep skillet over heat and add oil, vinegar, and a pinch of salt and pepper. Let sizzle for a few seconds and drizzle over fish with salsa. Serve immediately.

<u>Spicy Leek Meatballs</u>
4 servings

Notice that this recipe contains chili peppers. Select them based on how spicy or non-spicy you like your food. Chili peppers are high in magnesium, potassium, Vitamin C, and carotene.

1 lb. lean ground turkey or ground beef
1 ½ c. minced leeks (white and light green parts-about one bunch)
2 fresh chili peppers, minced
1 tbsp. fresh ginger, minced or 1 tsp. dried
2 tbsp. gluten-free flour
2 tbsp. sesame oil
Sea salt and pepper

Place all ingredients in a large mixing bowl. Knead by hand until ingredients are mixed.

Divide the mixture into 10-12 equal portions. Roll each into a ball (add a little flour to your hands if it is really sticky). Heat the oil in a large skillet over medium-high heat. Add meatballs and pan-fry, covered, turning occasionally, until browned on all sides and cooked through—about 10 minutes. Drain on a paper towel. Serve over steamed greens or any way you like. They can be frozen and put into soups also.

Awesome Grilled Salmon
Eight to ten 4 oz. servings

The ginger-lime marinade makes this dish really special. **NOTE:** One hour is needed for marinating before grilling.

1/3 c. tamari (This is dark soy sauce, and it can be found gluten-free and/or low salt if needed.)
2 tsp. toasted sesame oil
2 tbsp. grated ginger or 1 tsp. dried
Juice of 1 large lime
4 cloves garlic, minced
4 scallions, finely chopped
2-3 pounds salmon fillet (wild preferred)
2 red peppers, cut into chunks (optional)

Put tamari, oil, ginger, lime juice, garlic, and scallions in a small mixing bowl and whisk together. Place salmon in a shallow pan and pour the marinade on top. Allow to marinade for 1 hour in the refrigerator. Prepare the grill. When grill is hot, place the salmon on the grill, skin side down. Brush salmon with marinade and cook for 5 minutes. Turn salmon over and remove the skin. (It should come off easily.) Brush on marinade again and grill for 4-7 minutes until the thickest part is tender. Roast chunks of pepper on the grill while cooking salmon and serve alongside if desired.

Greek Shrimp Stew
6 servings

This is quick and easy to make. It can be served with gluten-free bread and a good salad.

1 tbsp. olive oil or coconut oil
2 onions, chopped
1 tsp. sea salt
4 cloves garlic, minced
3 c. chopped tomatoes
1 c. tomato sauce
2 tsp. Dijon mustard
3 tbsp. fresh dill, chopped or 1 tbsp. dried
1 tsp. honey
1 pound cooked shrimp
¼ - ½ c. feta cheese, crumbled
1 c. chopped fresh parsley

In a large pot, heat oil and add onions, salt, and garlic. Sauté until soft. Add tomatoes, tomato sauce, mustard, dill, and honey and simmer for 20 minutes on low heat. Five minutes before serving, add shrimp, feta, and parsley. Stir and serve.

Easy Stir-Fry
4-6 servings

You can follow this recipe with chicken or substitute non-GMO tofu, shrimp, or beef for variety. Try other veggie options like asparagus, shredded cabbage, snow peas, etc. It can be served over cooked brown rice, gluten-free pasta, or quinoa.

Sauce:
1 tbsp. cornstarch
½ c. chicken broth (or water)
1 tsp. honey or other healthy sweetener
1 tbsp. soy sauce
2 tbsp. peanut or sesame oil
2 garlic cloves, minced

Stir-Fry:
2 tbsp. coconut oil
1 pound chicken, thinly sliced
3 cups thinly sliced vegetables
(carrots, celery, onion, peppers, etc.)

Combine cornstarch and broth. Stir. Add remaining sauce ingredients until dissolved. Place a large skillet over high heat and add 1 tbsp. coconut oil. Stir-fry chicken for 3-4 minutes. Remove from skillet. Add the remaining oil and the longest cooking vegetables and stir-fry for 1 minute. Add remaining vegetables and cook until crisp and tender. Return chicken to skillet and add sauce. Stir until thick and serve.

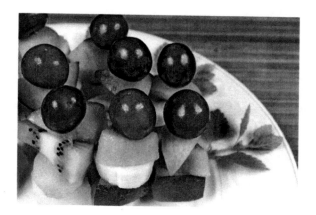

❖ Desserts (Yum!)

Everybody needs a little dessert once in a while to stay happy and satisfied. Don't overdo it, and don't punish yourself for eating it. (That's just destructive.) Besides, if you make healthy choices like the ones below, you'll be fine.

What We Love:

♥ Some of the sweet options listed under snacks.

♥ Dark chocolate

♥ Hodgson Mills Gluten-Free Brownie Mix

Yes, it contains some sugar, but much less than many other gluten-free baking mixes. (When you are shopping be diligent about checking for sugar content.) You can top these brownies with cut strawberries and a little real whipped cream. (Did you know that 2 tbsp. of whipped cream in the can only has 1 gram of sugar? Yum!!) These brownies can be purchased almost anywhere (http://www.hodgsonmillstore.com/en/gluten-free.aspx?p=2-12).

Gluten-Free Apple Crisp
4 servings

This is an easy-to-make recipe—even if you do not spend a lot of time in the kitchen. It uses coconut sugar, which is taken from the sap of the coconut palm blossom and tastes a little bit like molasses. It has a low glycemic value (won't elevate your body's blood sugar), and it can be substituted, 1 for 1, for any other sweetener. You may be able to locate it at Whole Foods, or you can get it online: http://www.essentiallivingfoods.com/low-glycemic-sweeteners/coconut-sugar.html.

Filling:
3-4 baking apples, cored, peeled, and sliced thin
2-4 tsp. honey or agave nectar
1 tbsp. arrowroot powder
1 tbsp. lemon juice
2 tsp. cinnamon

Topping:
1 ½ c. gluten-free rolled oats
½ c. sweet rice flour
½ -3/4 c. coconut sugar (or another natural sweetener of your choice)
1 tsp. cinnamon
¼ tsp. sea salt
½ c. melted coconut oil or butter
1 tsp. vanilla extract

Preheat oven to 375 degrees. Place all filling ingredients in a 7x11 baking pan (or sized close). Stir all together with a large spoon. Apples should come almost all the way to the top as they will cook down. In a small mixing bowl, stir oats, flour, sugar, cinnamon, and sea salt together. Add oil and vanilla, stirring together with a fork. Using your hands, crumble mixture on top of apple filling. Bake for 40 minutes or until juices are bubbling and the top is lightly browned.

Banana Nice Cream
2 servings

This is a really easy recipe to make. Double or triple the recipe, and you'll have leftovers. Peel, slice, and freeze bananas a day ahead so that they are ready.

2 bananas, peeled, sliced, and frozen
1 cup unsweetened vanilla almond milk
2 tbsp. smooth almond butter or peanut butter

Put all ingredients into a blender and puree. Shut motor off and stir 3-4 times until it is smooth and creamy. Put into 2 bowls and serve.

Coconut Macaroons
1 ½ dozen small cookies

These taste great, and they can be kept in the refrigerator in a sealed container for weeks. Don't eat them all at once!

1 tsp. coconut oil or butter for the baking sheet
3 c. shredded unsweetened coconut
1/3 c. coconut sugar or granulated stevia
Pinch of sea salt
3 large eggs
1 tsp. vanilla extract

Preheat oven to 350 degrees. Lightly oil the baking sheet with oil. Combine coconut, sugar, and salt in medium-sized bowl and mix well. In another bowl, place eggs and vanilla, whisking for about 3 minutes until the eggs are foamy. Mix eggs with coconut mixture and blend well. Drop by rounded teaspoons onto the baking sheet and bake for 15 minutes until they are golden on the top and edges. Gently take macaroons off of the sheet and place them on rack to cool.

Rice Pudding
6 servings

This is easy, and it takes about 20 minutes to prepare. It can be served warm or cold.

2 c. leftover brown or brown basmati rice
1 to 2 c. coconut water, almond milk, or non GMO soy milk
1 tsp. cinnamon
½ tsp. ground cardamom
½ c. raisins or dried fruit of your choice
½ c. shredded coconut
2 tbsp. honey or natural sweetener of your choice

Place all ingredients in a pot and bring to a boil. Reduce heat and simmer, stirring every couple of minutes. Continue cooking until dried fruit is plump; coconut is soft; and most of the liquid is gone. Taste and adjust spices if necessary. Serve or store in the refrigerator in an airtight container.

<u>Blueberries with Lemon Cream</u>
4 half cup servings

Add an extra teaspoon of lemon juice for great lemon flavor. Make sure you wash your blueberries with a veggie wash and let them dry on a towel before preparing.

4 oz. reduced fat or regular cream cheese, softened
¾ c. vanilla regular or Greek yogurt
1 tsp. honey or other natural sweetener
2 tsp. grated lemon zest
2 c. fresh blueberries

In a medium bowl, break up cream cheese with a fork and add yogurt and honey. If you have an electric mixer, beat until light and creamy. Otherwise, use a whisk and do it by hand. Add lemon zest and stir. Layer the cream cheese mixture, alternating with blueberries in dessert dishes or wine glasses. If you are not serving immediately, cover up to 8 hours in the refrigerator.

Almond Cream with Strawberries
4 servings

A little sweetened ricotta over berries for a happy tummy dessert in less than 10 minutes.

¼ c. sliced or slivered almonds
2 c. strawberries, washed, tops cut off and sliced
1 c. ricotta cheese
2 tbsp. all natural sweetener
¼ tsp. almond extract

Toast almonds in a dry skillet over medium heat. Stir until they are light brown and smell good. Transfer them to a plate to cool. Divide strawberries into 4 small serving dishes. Mix ricotta with almond extract and sweetener and mix until smooth. Spoon mixture over berries and sprinkle almonds on top. Serve.

Caramelized Bananas
2 servings

This recipe can easily be doubled for 4 people. The bananas cook in under 2 minutes so that they stay firm in the center.

2 medium firm bananas, peeled
½ tbsp. butter
3 tbsp. light brown sugar (ok as a treat)
¼ c. orange juice
1/8 tsp. cinnamon
1 c. healthy vanilla ice cream or yogurt

Cut bananas in half lengthwise. Heat butter in a medium sized skillet. Add brown sugar and mix with butter. Place bananas on top, cut side up. Cook without touching for 20-30 seconds. Add orange juice and cinnamon. Turn bananas gently and cook for 45-60 seconds more, basting with the sauce in the pan. Divide the bananas onto two plates and drizzle them with the sauce. Serve immediately with a small scoop of ice cream.

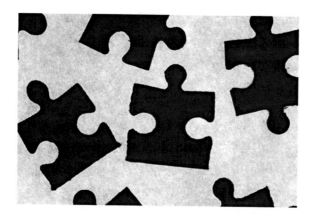

"In helping others, we shall help ourselves, for whatever good we give out completes the circle and comes back to us." - Flora Edwards

CONCLUSION

Watching my teenage son dealing with his Mild Traumatic Brain Injury on a daily basis has been both frustrating and very humbling as a parent. Besides keeping him in the forefront of my deepest prayers, there is not much that I can fix in his brain on my own. I have done and will continue to do what I do best; research and implement proven proactive ways, tools, and methods which will serve him as he steps THROUGH this journey to the healing side.

I have taken my Integrative Nutrition education and our experience of living with Mild Traumatic Brain Injury to serve you with this book and all of its helpful resources so that you do not have to navigate it all on your own. I hope that reading this book has allowed you to believe that you can be an advocate for your health and make educated decisions to further facilitate your healing as you progress, day by day, to increase your quality of life.

By following the information in this book, you can reduce the negative effects that poor food choices have on your brain, and you can promote healing and strength by adding whole foods, which will sustain your energy (and taste good, too!).

You will continue to have days that are tough and days when you feel great. Remember, it is okay to ask for help when you are tired, in pain, or just can't pull it together today. Allow people who care about you to give you emotional support and encourage them to accept who you are right now, even if some things have changed from the person you were before your injury.

God has a plan for you—even if you can't wrap your head around what the specifics of that plan might be right now. As I witness my son face each MTBI day with extreme bravery and courage, dealing with issues and symptoms that his peers have never even had to think about, I am excited to see how he is grabbing hold of new skills and even developing a more lighthearted sense of humor. Who knows how he will be called upon as he moves through the world with a mature level of compassion and innate strength. These attributes can never be taken away from him. I can't wait to see how his future unfolds.

I'm also looking forward to seeing how you will heal and grow in your future. Please share your story on my Facebook page – "Nourish Your Noggin!" or contact me through my website: www.nourishyournoggin.com . If you would like to explore my other offerings and individual and group coaching services, I welcome your inquiry at my website as well.

Wishing you the best,

Tina Sullivan
Integrative Health and Nutrition Coach, AADP, LLC
Contact me: support@nourishyournoggin.com

QUESTIONS?

Here Are Some Great Resources for You!

As a proactive advocate for my son and an Integrative Health and Nutrition Coach, it is my mission to learn about and locate both mainstream and alternative resources that may help to provide cutting edge information as well as therapies that may also hasten healing time. I have listed those organizations and websites here. I have also included nutritional websites as well. (Many of our favorite food manufacturers' websites have been listed throughout the previous chapters.) I hope that these resources help you to discover the many options that are available to you.

Nutrition Related Resources

Environmental Working Group (EWG):

http://www.ewg.org

This website contains information on the "Shoppers Guide to Pesticides in Produce."

Local Harvest:

http://www.localharvest.org/

Use this site to find local farmers markets, family farms, and other sustainable food options in your area.

Gluten Intolerance Group:

http://www.gluten.net/

This website contains information and education about gluten for individuals, families, and healthcare professionals.

Eat Well Guide:

http://www.eatwellguide.org/i.php?pd=Home

This is a free online directory of local food supplies, restaurants, and more.

Organic Consumers Association: http://www.organicconsumers.org/aboutus.cfm

This is an online grassroots and non-profit organization that deals with crucial issues of food safety, industrial agriculture, corporate accountability, and genetic engineering. This is a great website to find out what's really going on within the food and agriculture industry.

Institute for Integrative Nutrition: (This is where I went to school!) http://www.integrativenutrition.com/

Since 1992, Integrative Nutrition has been the cutting-edge leader in holistic nutrition education. As the largest nutrition school in the world, they educate and transform the lives of students with the world's foremost experts in nutrition and wellness, like Andrew Weil, MD, Arthur Agatston, MD, Barry Sears, PhD, Mark Hyman, MD and Geneen Roth, and many others. Their curriculum teaches a wide variety of skills in health coaching, nutrition education, business management, and healthy lifestyle choices.

Whole Foods:

http://www.wholefoodsmarket.com/

This is the world's largest retailer of natural and organic foods in North America. This is a great website for recipes, information, and to locate a store near you.

Trader Joe's:

http://www.traderjoes.com/

This is a specialty retail grocery store in many US states, and one of my favorite affordable retailers. Check their site to see if there is a store near you.

Living Without **Magazine:**

http://www.livingwithout.com/

This is a lifestyle guide for people with allergies and food sensitivities.

Eating Well Magazine:

http://www.eatingwell.com/

Look here for ideas for healthy eating, healthy cooking, and great recipes.

Neurological Resources

Center for Neuro Skills: http://www.neuroskills.com/mtbi.shtml

This particular page is all about Mild Traumatic Brain Injury, but this site has a huge amount of information, resources, and articles for you to check out.

Dr. Daniel Amen:

http://www.amenclinics.com/meet-dr-amen/

Dr. Amen is a physician, child and adult psychiatrist, and brain imaging specialist, and he has clinics in California, Washington State, and Reston, VA. He has created the Amen Solution, which is a way to overcome many physical obstacles in one's life by using the amazing power stored within your brain.

Dr. Stephen Kiraly, MD: http://www.healthybrain.org/home.html

He developed the Healthy Brain Program, and his business is based in Canada. He wrote the book, *Your Healthy Brain*.

Dr. Diane Roberts Stoler, Ed.D:

http://www.health-helper.com/

(This is my son's doctor.)

Dr. Diane Roberts Stoler is a neuropsychologist and a psychologist, who is Board Certified in Health and Sports Psychology. She specializes in Brain Rehabilitation Therapies and Brain Fitness for Athletes. She also wrote the very helpful book, *Coping with Mild Traumatic Brain Injury*.

Brain Injury Association of America: http://www.biausa.org/index.htm

This organization provides useful information, publications, and referrals to local chapters in support of individuals with brain injury, their families, and medical professionals.

Brain Line:

http://www.brainline.org/

This website contains information about preventing, treating, and living with TBI. This site highlights TBI topics, research updates, personal stories, and resource information for individuals, families, and professionals.

Traumatic Brain Injury:

http://www.traumaticbraininjury.com/

This website is dedicated to education, advocacy, legal guidance, and support for TBI survivors.

Wisconsin Sports Concussion Collaborative: http://www.wisportsconcussion.org/

This website and the collaborative effort that it represents are about creating a "safety net" for athletes by providing an easily accessible resource to help improve concussion education, identification, assessment, and management.

Traumatic Brain Injury Resource and Support Center: http://byyourside.org/

Based in Florida, this site is for athletes, coaches, parents, and trainers to learn about concussion and brain injuries. Their mission is to "inform," "support," "educate," and "advocate."

Sports Concussions: http://www.sportsconcussions.org/index.html

This helpful site was founded and created by Jean Rickerson, whose son suffered a Traumatic Brain Injury during a football game in 2008. She created this website to be a help for others and provide up-to-date research, news, and information to the public through this forum.

Sports Legacy Institute:

http://www.sportslegacy.org/

The mission of the Sports Legacy Institute is to advance the study, treatment, and prevention of the effects of brain trauma in athletes and other at-risk groups. In 2008, SLI partnered with the Boston University School of Medicine to form the Center for the Study of Traumatic Encephalopathy (CSTE). They also have developed ways to raise awareness of the issue and directly educate coaches, athletes, and parents.

Real Warriors:

http://www.realwarriors.net/

This is an initiative launched by the Defense Centers of Excellence for Psychological Health and Traumatic Brain Injury (DCoE) to promote the processes of building resilience, facilitating recovery and supporting reintegration of returning service members, veterans, and their families.

Defense and Veterans Brain Injury Center: http://www.dvbic.org/

Their mission is to serve active duty military, their beneficiaries, and veterans with traumatic brain injuries (TBIs) through state-of-the-art clinical care, innovative clinical research initiatives, and educational programs. DVBIC fulfills this mission through ongoing collaboration with military, VA and civilian health partners, local communities, families, and individuals with TBI.

Alternative Resources

Optometrists Network: http://www.braininjuries.org/brain_injury_double_vision.html

This is a helpful site that provides information regarding Post Traumatic Vision Syndrome, all of the symptoms that may be involved, what the options for treatment are, and places and doctors that provide it.

Neuro Optometric Rehabilitation Association: http://www.nora.cc/index.php

The Neuro-Optometric Rehabilitation Association, International (NORA) is a group of committed individuals from various disciplines focused on advancing the art and science of rehabilitation for the neurologically challenged patient. They provide resources and in depth information regarding vision issues after traumatic brain injury.

Vestibular Disorders Association: http://www.vestibular.org/index.php

This site provides information about balance issues, vertigo, dizziness, and other vestibular disorders. It explains symptoms and testing that may help to relieve symptoms.

American Chiropractic Board of Sports Physicians: http://www.acbsp.com/

This site's mission is to promote the highest standards of excellence and clinical competence for chiropractors specializing in sports medicine and physical fitness.

American Chiropractic Association:

http://www.acatoday.org/

The ACA is a professional organization representing Doctors of Chiropractic. It provides educational information and referrals to practitioners in your local area.

American Physical Therapy Association:

http://www.apta.org/

This site will provide you with information about physical therapy and lists physical therapists in your area.

National Association of Cognitive-Behavioral Therapists: http://www.nacbt.org/

The NACBT is the leading organization dedicated to supporting, promoting, teaching, and developing cognitive-behavioral therapy and those who practice it. Cognitive-behavioral therapy is effective in helping people make emotional and behavioral changes.

National Center for Homeopathy: http://nationalcenterforhomeopathy.org/

This organization provides educational information about homeopathic treatment and has a national directory of homeopaths.

CranioSacral Therapy: http://www.upledger.com/content.asp?id=26

CST is a gentle, hands-on method of evaluating and enhancing the functioning of a physiological body system called the craniosacral system, which is comprised of the membranes and cerebrospinal fluid that surround and protect the brain and spinal cord. This site provides a directory to local providers.

Reiki (Hands-on Healing):

http://www.reikienergy.com/

Reiki (Ray-Key) is an ancient, gentle, hands-on healing art that helps you feel better and heal better. Dr. Usui, a Japanese Christian educator, rediscovered this healing method in his study of ancient Tibetan texts. You can use Reiki to facilitate deep relaxation, relieve pain, and promote healing and personal growth. Reiki stimulates your body's innate healing resources, encouraging a return to wellness.

Electromagnetic Sensitivity:

http://www.earthcalm.com/emf-health-effects/electrosensitivity/

Electromagnetic Sensitivity is a new, but rapidly growing, disease. Electrosensitive people feel weakened or ill when around electromagnetic fields (EMFs). EMFs emanate from the electrical grid in buildings, all appliances, computers, and also from all wireless devices, such as cell phones and WiFi, as well as from cell towers and power lines. This site provides information, products, and research about this topic.

The Irlen Method:

http://irlen.com/index.php?s=index

Helen Irlen, MA, LMFT, the nation's leading expert in perceptually-based reading and learning difficulties, discovered and created the Irlen Method in 1980, and it is now being used in over 42 countries. This technology can improve reading fluency, comfort, comprehension, attention, and concentration, while reducing light sensitivity. This is not a method of reading instruction. It is a color-based technology that filters out offensive light waves so that the brain can accurately process visual information. For many, a traumatic brain injury (TBI) can result in significant sensitivity to light, glare, contrast, bright colors, patterns, and an inability to maintain attention and concentration. The Irlen Method can eliminate or improve these difficulties and improve the ability to function.

INDEX

BIBLIOGRAPHY

CHAPTER 1:

Kiraly, Stephen, MD, FRCPC, *Your Healthy Brain: A Personal & Family Guide to Staying Healthy & Living Longer*. Vancouver, B.C.Canada, Westcoast Reproductions, 2008. www.healthybrain. org, http://www.healthybrain.org/bookbibliography.html

Stoler, Diane Roberts, Ed.D, *Coping With Mild Traumatic Brain Injury: A Guide to Living with the Challenges Associated with Concussion/Brain Injury*. New York, NY, Avery, a member of Penguin Group, 1998. www.drdiane.com

www.ninds.nih.gov/disorders/tbi/detail_tbi.htm

www.traumaticbraininjury.com

http://www.cdc.gov/TraumaticBrainInjury/index.html

http://www.sportslegacy.org/

http://www.bu.edu/cste/

Chapter 2:

Adapted from, Phyllis A. Balch, CNC, *Prescription for Nutritional Healing*, Avery, NY, 2000.

http://www.fns.usda.gov/fdd/facts/nutrition/TransFatFactSheet. pdf

Allison Anneser, *Refined to Real Food*, Publishing Works, Inc., Exeter, NH, 2005.

Chapter 3:

http://www.huffingtonpost.com/dr-david-perlmutter-md/gluten-impacts-the-brain_b_785901.html

http://www.livingwithout.com/issues/1_11/untreated_gluten_ sensitivity-1800-1.html 1

http://glutenfreeville.com/featured/why-go-gluten-free

Dr. Mercola, *"This Common Food Ingredient Can Really Mess Up Your Metabolism,"* January 26, 2010.

http://ezinearticles.com/?Brain-Food---5-Foods-that-Nourish-the-Noggin&id=983003

http://healthypets.mercola.com/sites/articles/ archive/2010/01/02/HighFructose-Corn-Syrup-Alters-Human-Metabolism.aspx (full bibliography on this page)

Humphries P., Pretorius E., and Naude H., *"Direct and Indirect Cellular of Aspartame on the Brain,"* European Journal of Clinical Nutrition; 62(4):451-62 (April 2008).

Nutrition Research Newsletter. *"An artificial sweetener that can cause irreversible damage to your brain and body."* FindArticles.

com. 09 Feb, 2011.

Colbin, AnneMarie, *"Aspartame: The Real Story"* and *Integrative Nutrition-"Artificial Sweeteners,"* 2009.

Rosenthal, Joshua, *"Integrative Nutrition,"* Greenleaf Book Group LP, Austin, TX, 2008.

http://www.psychologytoday.com/blog/the-depression-cure/200907/dietary-sugar-and-mental-illness-surprising-link, *"The Depression Cure,"* Dr. Stephen Ilardi, PhD.

Willet, Walter, MD, *"Eat, Drink and Be Healthy: The Harvard Medical School Guide to Healthy Eating"* Free Press, 2002.

http://www.bantransfats.com/abouttransfat.html

http://www.cspinet.org/reports/chemcuisine.htm

http://msgtruth.org/body.htm

Kiraly,Stephen, MD, FRCPC, *"Your Healthy Brain: A Personal & Family Guide to Staying Healthy & Living Longer."* Vancouver, B.C., Canada, Westcoast Reproductions, 2008. www.healthybrain.org, http://www.healthybrain.org/bookbibliography.html

http://www.ewg.org/

Chapter 4:

http://www.healthynewage.com/blog/yacon-syrup/#ixzz1AHk2FgBd

http://nutritiondata.self.com/

Allison Anneser, *Refined to Real Food*, Publishing Works, Inc., Exeter, NH, 2005.

http://articles.mercola.com/sites/articles/archive/2010/10/22/coconut-oil-and-saturated-fats-can-make-you-healthy.aspx#_edn2

Dr. Mary G. Enig, Ph.D., F.A.C.N. <u>Source: Coconut: In Support of Good Health in the 21st Century, part 2.</u>

http://www.coconutoil.com/research.htm

http://coconutdiet.com/alzheimers.htm

http://www.blueocean.org/home

http://www.nongmoproject.org/consumers/about-gmos/

http://www.theamazingavocado.com/nutrition/benefits/

Rosenthal, Joshua, *"Integrative Nutrition,"* Greenleaf Book Group LP, Austin, TX, 2008.

http://www.wisegeek.com/what-is-palm-sugar.htm

http://www.amenclinics.com/cybcyb/foods-recipes/10-brain-healthy-spices/

Chapter 5:

Albi, Johnnna & Walthers, Catherine, *Greens, Glorious Greens!,*

New York: St. Martin's Press, 1996.

Allison Anneser, *Refined to Real Food*, Publishing Works, Inc., Exeter, NH, 2005.

http://www.wholefoodsmarket.com/recipes/2935

Beale, Lucy & Partridge, Jessica, *Eating Well on a Budget,* New York: Penguin Group, 2010.

Flay, Bobby. http://www.foodnetwork.com. 2010. Accessed 20 July 2010.

Lair, Cynthia. *Feeding the Whole Family.* Seattle: Sasquatch Books, 2008.

Rosenthal, Joshua, "*Integrative Nutrition*", Greenleaf Book Group LP, Austin, TX, 2008.

Savona, Natalie, *The Big Book of Juices And Smoothies,* London: Duncan Baird Publishers Ltd, 2003.

Watson, Brenda. *The Fiber 35 Diet.* New York: Free Press, A Division of Simon & Schuster, Inc., 2007.

Willett, Walter, M.D. and Katzen, Mollie, *Eat, Drink & Weigh Less,* New York: Hyperion, 2006.

Yeager, Selene. *The Doctors Book of Food Remedies.* Emmanus, Pennsylvania: Rodale Press, 1998.

"Banana Nice Cream Snack". http://www.wholefoodsmarket.com/

recipes/2739. 2011. Accessed 14 June 2011.

"Apple Sandwiches". http://www.wholefoodsmarket.com/recipes/2535. 2011. Accessed 15 June 2011.

"Quick and Spicy Tamari Nut Mix". http://www.wholefoodsmarket.com/recipes/80 2011. Accessed 15 June 2011.

"Gluten-Free Chex Style Mix". http://glutenfreecooking.about.com/od/appetizerssnacksand/r/gfchexstylemix.htm. 2011. Accessed 14 June 2011.

"Gluten-Free Apple Crisp". http://www.nourishingmeals.com/2009/09/coconut-sugar-apple-crisp-and-giveaway.html. 2011. Accessed on 15 June 2011.

"Blueberries and Lemon Cream." http://www.eatingwell.com/recipes/blueberries_with_lemon_cream.html. 2003. Accessed 15June 2011.

"Almond Cream with Strawberries." http://www.eatingwell.com/recipes/almond_cream_with_strawberries.html. March 1998. Accessed 15 June 2011.

"Caramelized Bananas." http://www.eatingwell.com/recipes/caramelized_bananas.html 2004. Accessed 16 June 2011.

ABOUT THE AUTHOR

Tina Sullivan currently resides in New Hampshire with her husband and two sons.

Earlier in her life, Tina Sullivan received National Certification as an Ultrasound Technologist from the University of Medicine & Dentistry in Newark, New Jersey, where she was educated on how the body works in depth.

In addition to being certified by the American Association of Drugless Practitioners, Tina Sullivan has been trained in a multitude of nutritional theories, from Ayurvedic to Macrobiotic to the Zone diet and almost everything in between. She's been taught by leading natural health and nutrition experts, such as Dr. Andrew Weil, Deepak Chopra, Dr. Walter Willet from Harvard, Geneen Roth and many others. Through the Institute of Integrative Nutrition in New York City, New York, she has become a Certified Integrative Health & Nutrition Coach.

Here are some of Tina's certifications, memberships, and degrees that you should know about:

- **Certified Integrative Health & Nutrition Coach, AADP,** Institute of Integrative Nutrition, NYC

- **Ultrasound Technologist, School of Health Related Professions,** University of Medicine & Dentistry

- **Integrative Practitioner Member**, leading online community for practitioners of Integrative Medicine

- **Holistic Practitioners of New Hampshire**, member

- **Manchester Holistic Health Examiner**, for "Examiner.com" an online National e-zine (published author)

This training has proven to be a wonderful reflection on the successes of her clients, as they have made tremendous strides in their food and lifestyle choices that work best for their unique needs.

For more information about individual and group coaching services, or to explore other product offerings available to you, please visit her website: www.nourishyournoggin.com or email her at support@nourishyournoggin.com